**This book is to be returned on or before
the last date stamped below.**

Ph

a se

Gener

Dr R
Physi

Prof
Depa
Midc

Prof
Depa
Hosp

Dis

11242

HOBSLEY, Michael

WI
100

Physiological Principles in Medicine:

Books are published in linked pairs—the preclinical volume linked to its clinical counterpart, as follows:

Endocrine Physiology by Richard N. Hardy
Clinical Endocrinology by Peter Daggett

Digestive System Physiology by Paul A. Sanford
Disorders of the Digestive System by Michael Hobsley

In preparation:

The Physiology of Respiration by John Widdicombe and Andrew Davies
Respiratory Disorders by Ian R. Cameron

Disorders of the Digestive System

Michael Hobsley TD, PhD, MChir, FRCS

Professor of Surgical Science, The Middlesex Hospital Medical School, London

Edward Arnold

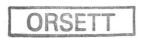

First published 1982
by Edward Arnold (Publishers) Ltd.
41 Bedford Square, London WC1B 3DQ

British Library Cataloguing in Publication Data
Hobsley, M.
Disorders of the Digestive System. –
(Physiological principles in medicine).
1. Digestive organs – Diseases
I. Title   II. Series
616.3   RC801
ISBN 0-7131-4381-9
ISSN 0260-2946

Filmset in Compugraphic Baskerville by
Reproduction Drawings Ltd., Sutton, Surrey
and printed in Great Britain by
Spottiswoode Ballantyne Ltd., Colchester and London

General preface to series

Student textbooks of medicine seek to present the subject of human diseases and their treatment in a manner that is not only informative, but interesting and readily assimilable. It is also important, in a field where knowledge advances rapidly, that the principles are emphasized rather than details, so that information remains valid for as long as possible.

These factors all favour an approach which concentrates on each disease as a disturbance of normal structure and function. Therapy, in principle, follows logically from a knowledge of the disturbance, though it is in this field that the most rapid changes in information occur.

A disturbance of normal structure without any disturbance of function is not important to the patient except for cosmetic or psychological considerations. Therefore, it is the disturbance in function which should be stressed. Preclinical students must get a firm grasp of physiology in a way that shows them how it is related to disease, while clinical students must be presented with descriptions of disease which stress the basic disturbance of function that is responsible for symptoms and signs. This approach should increase interest, reduce the burden on the student's memory and remain valid despite alterations in the details of treatment, so long as the fundamental physiological concepts remain unchallenged.

In the present Series, the major physiological systems are each covered by a pair of books, one preclinical and one clinical, in which the authors have attempted to meet the requirements discussed above. A particular feature is the provision of cross-references between the two members of a pair of books to facilitate the blending of basic science and clinical expertise that is the goal of this Series.

RNH
MH
KBS

Preface

The approach adopted in this book to disorders of the digestive system is in terms of clinical situation rather than of individual diseases. Common clinical situations such as jaundice or disturbances of defaecation are presented and the student is shown how the experienced clinician analyses the problem and decides on management. Nevertheless, information on any disease can easily be looked up by reference to the index.

Terminology is always a problem for students embarking on a new field, and the clinical scene is no exception. In some curricula students have already studied pathology before coming to the wards, and they should have little difficulty. For the rest, the problem is greater. I have tried to mitigate the difficulty by explaining terms the first time they are used in the text, but a good medical dictionary will be very helpful.

A specific area where terminology can be particularly confusing is drugs: generic names and commonly used trade names may both change from one area of the English-speaking world to another. In general, the generic name in the UK is given in the text, sometimes with a commonly used UK trade name in parentheses; a list of all preparations mentioned is given in the Appendix, with US equivalents.

The general philosophy of the Series, that clinical matters will be described in the light of our knowledge of the underlying disturbances of physiology, has been closely followed in this book. In a few areas, such as gastric secretion in Chapter 4 and gastric emptying in Chapter 5, more details of tests of function are given than is usual in a text meant for clinical medical students, but it is hoped that these will help to illustrate the importance of physiological concepts and measurements in treating some patients. There has been the closest co-operation between Dr Paul Sanford, the author of the companion volume on the physiology of the digestive tract in this Series, and myself during the writing of the pair of books, and there are frequent cross-references in both texts to the companion volume.

Acknowledgements

It is a pleasure to thank my colleagues at The Middlesex Hospital for their help in criticizing the text and providing radiological, clinical and pathological illustrations, and in particular my medical gastroenterological colleague

Dr Peter Cotton. Specific sources are acknowledged in the captions, but I specially wish to thank Dr Brian Thomas of University College Hospital, London, for Fig. 2.2 and Dr John Olney of the Royal Free Hospital, London, for Fig. 6.4.

Miss Alison Thomson nobly bore the brunt of the burden of typing and retyping, and I am grateful to her for her efficiency and endurance!

I greatly appreciate the help given me by the publishers at all stages of the writing and production of this book.

Finally, to my wife and children for whom this book was yet another task that reduced my time with them, I express my gratitude for their forbearance.
1981   MH

Contents

1

Salivary glands

Although the secretion of the salivary glands initiates the process of digestion, disorders of these glands are not always considered to be the province of the gastroenterologist. Many other specialists, including general surgeons, otorhinolaryngologists, immunologists and plastic surgeons as well as general physicians, may find themselves treating diseases of the glands; numerically, the majority of patients require surgical attention. In terms of physiological systems, the digestive seems the best one under which to consider disorders of the salivary glands.

Symptoms of dysfunction

Patients whose major presenting complaint falls under this heading include those with a dry mouth and those with excessive salivation. The overwhelming majority of patients with either complaint show no evidence on examination of the mouth to substantiate their symptom; the impartial observer reckons that the dryness, or the obvious salivation, is within the rather wide spectrum of the normal range.

It is useful to have an objective test of the rate of salivary secretion. The best standardized appears to be Curry's, in which secretion from each parotid gland is collected (Sanford: *Digestive System Physiology*, Chapter 2) for 5 minutes after an intravenous injection of 5 mg pilocarpine nitrate, a dose that evokes maximum secretion. The normal range is 3–13 ml of secretion from each gland; patients with a secretion within this range and with no other evidence of disease of the salivary glands can be reassured that their subjective sensation of an abnormality in either direction has no organic basis and must be due to increased awareness of sensation in the oral mucosa. After such reassurance the symptoms usually diminish. The rare patients with a true reduction in secretion are likely to have some form of Sjögren's syndrome (p. 3), while hypersecretion with parotid glands visibly larger than normal has been described but is extremely rare.

Lump in parotid region

The boundaries of the parotid region are shown in Fig. 1.1. A swelling, not arising in skin, and which lies in or overlaps the boundary may be an intrinsic lesion of the salivary gland or may arise in some other structure such as a lymph node or the subcutaneous tissue. However, the chances are 3 : 1 that it is a neoplasm of the parotid itself. Three-quarters of parotid neoplasms are a benign lesion called *pleomorphic salivary adenoma* (the old name, which should be abandoned, was *mixed tumour*); however, this tumour and most other benign salivary tumours show an unpleasant tendency to recur locally as multiple seedling deposits if cells of the growth are shed into the tissues by a preliminary biopsy or during the process of removal. Because these benign lesions show also a distinct tendency to undergo malignant change as the years pass, the logical management of a subcutaneous lump in the parotid region is *complete excision-biopsy*; that is, removal of the lump with a wide margin of normal tissue and without any preliminary biopsy. This policy can be technically difficult because of the facial nerve trunk and its branches that lie within the gland and may be in very close proximity to the tumour, and in an ideal world the surgeon should have special training, experience and interest in this field. The operation is called *conservative parotidectomy* (because it

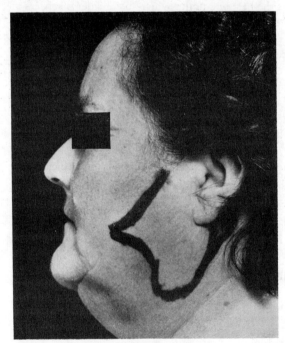

Fig. 1.1 This patient's left parotid salivary gland was indurated (because of Sjögren's disease, p. 3); its margins were easily identified and have been mapped with a skin pencil. Note how far downwards into the neck, and backwards over the mastoid process, the lower pole extends. The extension forwards along the parotid duct is called the accessory lobe.

conserves the facial nerve), and may be *superficial* if the lump is in that part of the gland superficial to the nerve, or *total* if the lump is found to be in the part deep to the nerve so that this part must be removed as well. Section of the facial nerve results in permanent paralysis of one-half of the face—an unpleasant deformity.

Malignant tumours of the parotid gland constitute about 10 per cent of all parotid tumours. They may give rise to a clinical suspicion of malignancy because of aggressively rapid growth or because of fixity to bone; such patients have a poor prognosis, fewer than 10 per cent being alive 5 years after diagnosis, and their management is an unsolved problem but usually involves some combination of surgery and radiotherapy. Sometimes a lump presenting without features of malignancy, and removed with a margin according to the policy of the previous paragraph, is reported by the histopathologist as being more malignant than expected, but the prognosis is substantially better in those cases. Occasionally, during what the surgeon embarked on as a conservative parotidectomy, he finds that the lump appears to be infiltrating one or more branches or even the trunk of the facial nerve rather than pushing them aside. In order to maintain the margin of normal tissue around the tumour, it is then necessary to sacrifice the whole nerve (*radical*) or one or more branches (*semi-conservative parotidectomy*).

Chronic or recurrent bilateral parotid swelling

The characteristic shape (Fig. 1.1) of the parotid salivary gland is maintained if the gland as a whole enlarges and becomes indurated because of chronic or recurrent disease. Recurrent attacks of acute pain and swelling are usually diagnosed as mumps in the first attack, but this diagnosis has to be reviewed when the attacks recur or if the glands remain persistently enlarged and hard.

This group of patients has not yet been well studied, but it would appear that many show in biopsy specimens the characteristic histological features of *Sjögren's disease* (syn. *benign lymphoepithelial disease*): infiltration with small round cells and proliferation of the ordinary epithelial cells and also the myoepithelial cells (Sanford: *Digestive System Physiology*, Chapter 2) of the parotid ducts, which may proceed to a degree that obliterates the lumen of the ducts. A few of these patients have other clinical features of the group constituting *Sjögren's syndrome*: dryness of the mouth (hyposecretion may be confirmed by Curry's test), dryness of the eyes (due to interstitial keratitis) and various rheumatic manifestations. Two-thirds of the patients have abnormal autoantibodies in their blood, including antibodies to salivary glands. The characteristic radiological finding in Sjögren's disease is punctate sialectasis (Fig. 1.2).

Apart from the suggestion that this is a disease of autoimmunity, little is known about its aetiology. It occurs at any age, and in infants and young adults is usually self-limiting after running a course of several years. Very rarely, some form of non-Hodgkin's lymphoma may develop.

Treatment is restricted to reassurance that in most patients the disease will 'burn itself out', although a few cases respond to large doses of steroids. Occasionally the symptoms are severe enough to warrant parotidectomy.

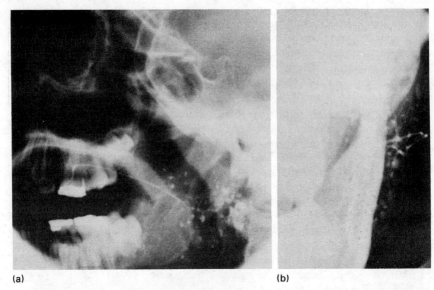

(a)   (b)

Fig. 1.2 Sialogram showing punctate sialectasis: (a) lateral view, and (b) anteroposterior view. The large ducts are normal (note how narrow these normal ducts are), but the walls of the finer ducts at their terminations are weakened by the disease so that the contrast material readily bursts through them to extravasate as globules.

A rare cause of chronic bilateral parotid swelling is *sarcoidosis*. Drugs such as *iodides* and anti-Parkinsonism agents, and malnutrition are other possible causes, although the mechanisms involved are unknown.

Chronic or recurrent unilateral parotid swelling

One-fifth of patients presenting in this category prove to be cases of Sjögren's disease in which the clinical symptoms are limited to one side, although punctate sialectasis can usually be demonstrated in the opposite parotid as well and in many patients the symptoms ultimately become bilateral. Most of the remaining four-fifths of patients probably have their bouts of painful parotid swelling due to the presence of a stone in the parotid duct, producing periodic impaction and obstruction with proximal sequestration of parotid secretion.

A careful history often distinguishes between Sjögren's disease and parotid duct calculus. In Sjögren's disease the attacks of swelling start gradually, last several days and fade gradually away, while dryness of the mouth is a chronic feature not particularly related to the attack in time or lateralized to the side of the attack. By contrast, the patient with a calculus says his attacks are sudden in onset and in ending, he is sometimes aware that the half of his mouth on the side of the affected gland is dry during the attack, the relief of symptoms is often ushered in by a gush of saliva into the mouth on the affected side, and the duration of the whole episode ranges from a few hours to a day or two at the most. Pain tends to be more intense in the shorter attacks with a stone than in the longer episodes of Sjögren's disease.

Inspection and palpation of Stensen's duct, particularly at its termination in the mouth opposite the second molar tooth, may confirm the presence of a stone or localized inflammation or deformation due to impaction of the stone. Radiology is always necessary to confirm the site and size of the stone because these factors determine treatment. Plain x-rays, particularly the anteroposterior and intrabuccal views (Fig. 1.3), may show the stone;

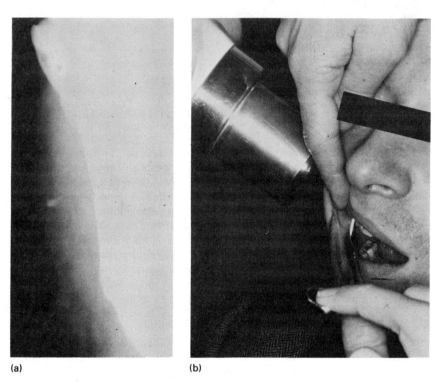

(a)   (b)

Fig. 1.3 (a) Plain x-ray, anteroposterior view, of the parotid region, showing a radio-opaque calculus. (b) Technique for obtaining an intrabuccal view of the termination of the parotid duct. This procedure eliminates the jaws and teeth from the background.

however, it may be very small (the calibre of the normal parotid duct is less than 1 mm) and radiolucent, so it is important to use sialography—the injection of a radio-opaque contrast medium into the duct system of a salivary gland via its oral orifice (Fig. 1.4). The calculus usually expresses itself as dilatation of the main duct system proximal to a filling defect or an apparent stricture, but occasionally produces a complete cut-off appearance of the main duct. These appearances are very different from the 'punctate sialectasis' of Sjögren's disease (see Fig. 1.2).

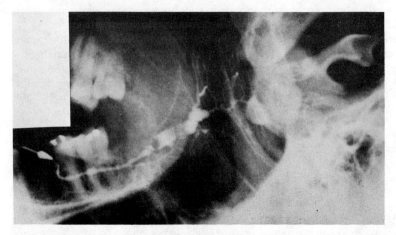

Fig. 1.4 Sialogram showing a stone in the parotid duct. The narrow calibre of the anterior segment, the rounded filling defect and the dilated posterior segment are well seen.

If the calculus is palpable at the oral orifice of the duct, or there is evidence that it has been impacted at that orifice, the opening of the duct should be enlarged by an operation via the mouth (*ductoplasty* or *duct meatotomy*). The same operation may be worth performing if the stone is impacted within 2 cm of the orifice, since this procedure may facilitate passage of the stone the next time it travels forwards and impacts. Stones further back should in the first instance be treated expectantly: certainly stones up to 3 mm in diameter are very likely to pass spontaneously. Larger stones require surgical removal, if the severity and frequency of the attacks warrant this. Even if the site of the stone can be determined because it is palpable in the cheek, cutting down on the stone is a hazardous procedure because of the close proximity to the duct of the two buccal branches of the facial nerve: these branches may wind round the duct at the anterior border of the masseter muscle and are then at great risk of being cut. Certainly if the stone is impalpable, the operation of superficial conservative parotidectomy is necessary, removing a long length of duct with its contained stone in continuity with the salivary gland.

Acute parotid swelling

Whether it is unilateral or bilateral, acute painful parotid swelling is usually diagnosed as mumps. Sometimes there are features that make the diagnosis virtually certain; for example, associated orchitis or pancreatitis, concurrence with an epidemic, or exposure to a contact with mumps 10–14 days earlier. The diagnosis can be confirmed by finding a rising titre of mumps antibody in the patient's serum, but it is not usually considered necessary to perform this investigation. Nearly always the attack subsides spontaneously and there is never any recurrence. This in itself can be taken as confirmation of the diagnosis, although presumably in some unilateral cases the cause was a stone that passed spontaneously at the first attempt!

A mechanical disturbance of drainage from the parotid duct orifice occasionally stems from a local lesion such as inflammation and oedema of a socket following tooth extraction; ascending infection can also be precipitated by poor oral hygiene in a debilitated patient, but this latter cause is rare in centres where nursing standards are high.

Disorders of submandibular salivary gland

The common affection of this salivary gland is a syndrome of recurrent bouts of painful swelling of one gland due to obstruction of its duct by a calculus. The attacks usually come on during a meal, when salivation increases, and subside within a few hours. The shorter duration, compared with symptoms due to a parotid duct calculus, may be due to the fact that impaction is less likely to be firm in the submandibular duct, of which the internal diameter is much greater than that of the parotid duct. The stone may be easily palpable in the duct in the floor of the mouth, or occasionally, if it is large and has impacted at the very beginning of the duct at the hilus of the gland, it may be felt via the neck. Nearly all submandibular calculi are radio-opaque and plain x-rays, particularly an intraoral view of the floor of the mouth (Fig. 1.5), usually confirm the diagnosis; occasionally sialography is necessary. A stone in the duct can be removed via a small incision through the wall of the duct and the overlying mucosa of the floor of the mouth, but a stone in the gland or

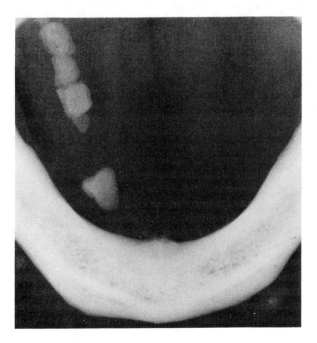

Fig. 1.5 Plain x-ray: intraoral view of floor of mouth, showing several radio-opaque stones in the submandibular duct near its orifice.

a gland that has become chronically infected and remains indurated between acute attacks requires removal of the whole salivary gland via a cervical incision.

All the neoplasms that occur in the parotid can also occur in the submandibular salivary gland. The absolute incidence of all the neoplasms is lower, but the proportion of malignant tumours is higher in the submandibular than in the parotid. In a patient with a palpable swelling in the submandibular region, failure of clinical and radiological examination to reveal a calculus in the gland or its duct suggests that a tumour is present, and an excision via the neck of the whole salivary gland with a wide margin of surrounding normal tissue is indicated.

Further reading

Conley, J. (1975). *Salivary Glands and the Facial Nerve.* Georg Thieme, Stuttgart.

Hobsley, M. (1973). Salivary tumours. *British Journal of Hospital Medicine* **10**, 553–562.

Stevens, K. L. H. and Hobsley, M. (1981). The treatment of pleomorphic adenoma by formal parotidectomy. *British Journal of Surgery* In press.

Suleiman, S. I., Thomson, J. P. S. and Hobsley, M. (1979). Recurrent unilateral swelling of the parotid gland. *Gut* **20**, 1102–1108.

Thackray, A. C. and Lucas, R. B. (1972). Tumors of the major salivary glands. *Atlas of Tumor Pathology,* Second Series, Fascicle 10. Armed Forces Institute of Pathology, Washington DC.

2

Oesophagus

The predominant symptom associated with oesophageal disease is *dysphagia*, a term which means difficulty in swallowing. Notice particularly that the difficulty is not necessarily pain. Moreover, localization by the subject of the site of his symptom is poor so that a complaint that the food seems to stick behind the lower end of the sternum, for example, is not good evidence that the obstruction is at the lower end of the oesophagus.

Spasm of the muscle of the oesophageal wall produces pain which is characteristically retrosternal and may radiate down the left arm, thus mimicking the pain of myocardial ischaemia. This symptom, independent of dysphagia, is a rare form of presentation of oesophageal disease.

Heartburn is discussed in Chapter 3.

There are no other *direct* symptoms of oesophageal disease, but symptoms due to secondary effects or related causes are considered below.

Dysphagia

History

A patient with dysphagia due to an organic constricting lesion in his gullet classically complains that at first the difficulty occurs only with solid foods which require considerable chewing, but that as time passes the difficulty increases until in the end liquids cannot be swallowed and the patient is in the pitiable state of being unable even to swallow his own saliva.

This relentless progression is typical of a neoplastic lesion. Other organic lesions such as inflammatory stricture or the muscular inco-ordination of achalasia (p. 12) may wax and wane in bouts superimposed on a generally downhill but sometimes only very slowly progressive course. Dysphagia can also be a symptom of neurosis, but then is typically worse with liquids than with solids.

The cause of the dysphagia is sometimes suggested by particular features of the history. The typical association with heartburn related to posture in patients with gastro-oesophageal reflux is discussed in Chapter 3; a history of swallowing corrosive liquids points to the dysphagia being due to a long fibrous cicatricial stricture. Acute inflammatory conditions of the mouth or pharynx may be obviously responsible, while the symptoms of a pharyngeal pouch (p. 11) are characteristic—the patient develops increasing dysphagia during a meal and may be aware of gurgling noises in his throat or neck, but after spontaneous or induced retching to empty the pouch by regurgitation he may be able to undertake a second instalment of the meal.

The consequences of dysphagia sometimes figure prominently in the history as weight loss and recurrent bouts of chest infections. The latter are due to the difficulty in swallowing causing food or saliva to enter the respiratory passages, whereupon localized or diffuse inflammation or bronchopulmonary segmental collapse may ensue.

Physical signs

The cervical oesophagus is almost completely protected from the clinician's sight and touch by the trachea in front and the spine behind; the thoracic oesophagus is even more remote. Thus physical signs related to the cause of the dysphagia are not often available. Occasionally there is evidence of an inflammatory lesion at or near the upper end of the oesophagus—pharyngitis, tonsillitis, retropharyngeal abscess or, rarely, acute thyroiditis; or a pharyngeal pouch may be palpable.

Associated aetiological and consequential factors are more likely to give rise to physical signs. The iron deficiency of *sideropenic dysphagia* (p. 11) may have resulted in anaemia with pallor of the mucous membranes and koilonychia (spoon-shaped nails) and often a sore, red tongue. The reduction in intake of food may have produced obvious evidence of loss of weight with emaciation, while if the difficulty has embraced liquids there may be evidence of dehydration or extracellular fluid depletion (page 116), depending on whether the lack is of water alone or of water and sodium chloride. Palpable cervical lymph nodes may result from metastatic spread of carcinoma of the oesophagus; this is a rare phenomenon, but palpable supraclavicular nodes are less uncommon when the primary lesion is a carcinoma of the cardiac region of the stomach involving the lower end of the oesophagus and thereby causing dysphagia. Spillage of oesophageal contents into the bronchial tree may have produced abnormal signs in the chest.

Investigations

A blood count reveals iron-deficiency anaemia by its microcytosis and hypochromia, with associated low values of the numerical indices of mean corpuscular volume (MCV) and mean corpuscular haemoglobin concentration (MCHC). Sometimes these overt changes have not yet developed, but an incipient iron deficiency can be uncovered by measurements of the plasma free iron concentration and the iron-binding capacity. Biochemical evidence of water and electrolyte depletion may also be available in blood and urine samples. However, the crucial investigation in patients with dysphagia is the so-called barium swallow: the patient swallows a few mouthfuls of a suspension of a barium salt, and a radiologist follows the passage of the opaque meal down the oesophagus by direct observation on a fluoroscopic screen and by taking still radiographs at intervals to record moments of particular interest. In some special centres a cinematographic record is also made.

If the barium swallow is normal, the chance that any serious abnormality of the oesophagus is present is so small that it is usually reasonable to reassure the patient. However, if there is any abnormality, or if the clinician has a high index of suspicion because of other circumstances in the particular case, or if the dysphagia persists despite reassurance after a normal barium swallow, then endoscopic examination with biopsy of any suspected lesion is indicated. The old, rigid oesophagoscopes are more dangerous with respect to perforating the oesophagus, but perhaps give a better view and a better chance of an accurate biopsy, than the modern flexible gastroscopes.

Finally, measurements of the high pressure zone (HPZ) of the lower (o)esophageal sphincter (LOS or LES) (Sanford: *Digestive System Physiology*, Chapter 2) can be helpful in dealing with patients with gastro-oesophageal reflux and/or hiatus hernia (p. 30), but are available only in special centres.

There now follows a description of the principal oesophageal diseases and their management.

Sideropenic dysphagia
(syn. (UK) Paterson–Brown–Kelly syndrome
  (USA) Plummer–Vinson syndrome)

This is a condition particularly of middle-aged women in which iron deficiency coexists with dysphagia. The link is unexplained, but the immediate cause of the dysphagia seems to be a mucosal fold (usually called a web) seen in the uppermost region of the oesophagus (behind the cricoid cartilage) as an anterior indentation of the opaque meal during the early phase of a barium swallow examination. Oesophagoscopy destroys the web and cures the dysphagia. The anaemia is sometimes refractory to oral iron, so intravenous or intramuscular injections may be needed.

The real importance of this condition is that it seems to predispose towards carcinoma of the postcricoid region of the pharyngo-oesophagus. The extent to which this predisposition is affected by correction of the anaemia is unclear.

Pharyngeal pouch
(syn. Pharyngeal diverticulum)

This is a herniation of mucous membrane from the posterior wall of the upper end of the oesophagus through a defect in the muscular wall of the pharyngo-oesophagus (Killian's dehiscence) at the upper border of the cricopharyngeus muscle (Fig. 2.1). As the pouch enlarges it deviates to one side of the neck or the other (usually the left) and ultimately presents in the anterior triangle of the neck at the junction of the upper and middle thirds of the sternomastoid muscle. Cinematographic studies suggest that an important aetiological factor is spasm of the cricopharyngeus muscle, which fails to relax as it should when

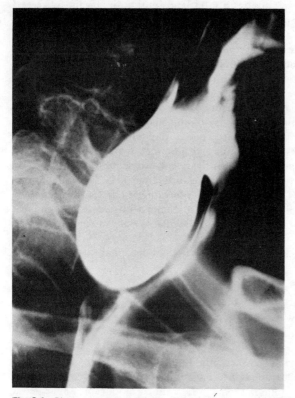

Fig. 2.1 Pharyngeal pouch. The swallowed barium has partly entered the sac. The production of dysphagia by obstruction of the upper end of the oesophagus as the sac enlarges is easily understood.

a bolus of food is delivered to that region by the act of swallowing, thus producing a sharp rise in the local intraluminal pressure (Sanford: *Digestive System Physiology*, Chapter 1).

The only effective treatment is surgical excision of the pouch via a cervical incision, and it is probably wise to divide the cricopharyngeus muscle at the neck of the hernia.

Achalasia of the oesophagus

This condition used to be called, inaccurately, achalasia of the cardia. There is no abnormality of the cardia: the abnormality lies in the lower end of the oesophagus, which fails to relax as a bolus of food reaches it. Achalasia is a word invented from Greek roots to express this lack of co-ordination.

The disorder is commonly very chronic: it may be many years before the first minor symptoms of dysphagia progress sufficiently to be a real nuisance to the patient. This extended time-scale gives opportunity to the oesophagus to dilate and hypertrophy above the region of obstruction. In the most severe cases the oesophagus also elongates and chronically contains a semi-solid mixture of oropharyngeal secretions and solid and liquid food. It may then be visible on a plain radiograph of the chest as a tortuous mediastinal shadow (Fig. 2.2), sometimes containing a fluid level.

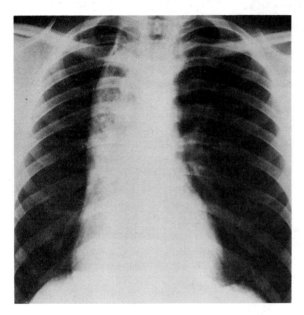

Fig. 2.2 Achalasia of the oesophagus. This chest x-ray shows two typical (though not invariable) features of advanced achalasia: the vertical opacity of the dilated oesophagus lying to the right of the denser shadow of the heart and aorta, and the absence of the gas/liquid level normally seen in the fundus of the stomach.   (X-ray kindly provided by Dr Brian Thomas, University College Hospital, London.)

The barium swallow (Fig. 2.3a) also demonstrates the grossly dilated proximal oesophagus; the lower end, though essentially normal in calibre, may by contrast be misinterpreted by the unwary as a stricture. The zone of junction between the proximal dilated and distal lower end is usually smooth and funnel-shaped, in contradistinction to the typical appearances of a carcinoma of the lower end of the oesophagus (p. 16; Fig. 2.3b). However, no matter how typical of achalasia the clinical and radiological features seem to be, the clinician should always proceed as though he were trying to confirm that the correct diagnosis is carcinoma: endoscopy and biopsy of the lower end of the oesophagus are mandatory, not just on one occasion, but freely repeated if there is any difficulty in collecting the tissue or interpreting the histological appearances, or if there is any definite change in the symptoms or signs of an established case of achalasia. Not only are the radiological appearances of a carcinoma sometimes confusingly similar to those of achalasia, but achalasia itself has been shown to predispose to carcinoma of the oesophagus.

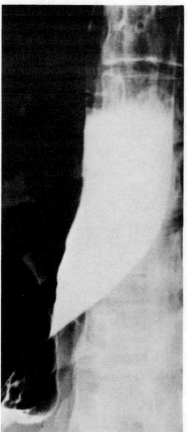

Fig. 2.3 Barium swallow appearances of (a) achalasia of the oesophagus, and (b) carcinoma of the lower third of the oesophagus. Note the smooth, funnel-shaped lower end to the dilated oesophagus in (a), and the ragged filling defect with 'shoulders' in (b).

(a)

(b)

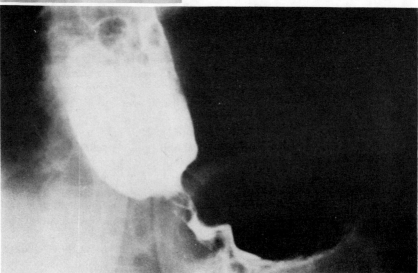

Achalasia is associated with a reduction in the number of ganglion cells in the extensive nerve plexuses of the lower oesophagus (Sanford: *Digestive System Physiology*, Chapter 2). In Europe and North America the cause is usually unknown, but in South America schistosomiasis (Chapter 6) is a common cause of destruction of ganglion cells of the oesophagus, and a similar picture of obstruction results (Chagas' disease).

Treatment

Many patients can be kept reasonably comfortable for many years by repeatedly stretching the lower end of the oesophagus with peroral dilators. Dilatation is first undertaken by passing a bougie via an oesophagoscope, and this procedure may be repeated at intervals; a few patients learn to swallow a bougie by their own efforts, but it is important to check by radiological screening that the bougie passes into the stomach rather than being accommodated in a cul-de-sac of the tortuous oesophagus. More forceful endoscopic dilatation has recently been introduced; it probably has the same mechanical effect as operation.

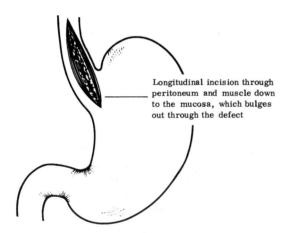

Longitudinal incision through peritoneum and muscle down to the mucosa, which bulges out through the defect

Fig. 2.4   Heller's operation or cardiomyotomy for achalasia of the cardia.

Operative treatment is usually more satisfactory. The procedure is known, after its inventor, as Heller's operation or cardiomyotomy (Fig. 2.4): a long incision is made through the muscle of the lower oesophagus in a vertical direction, and is prolonged for several centimetres downwards past the cardia into the upper end of the stomach. This incision divides all the muscular fibres but leaves intact the mucosa of the oesophagus and stomach which pouts through the muscular gap. This destroys the ability of the non-relaxing lower oesophagus to hold up the bolus, but at the cost of also destroying the valvular mechanism in this region which prevents reflux of acid–pepsin (and sometimes bile) from the stomach into the oesophagus (p. 24). However, the patients usually find that the improvement in swallowing outweighs the subsequent tendency to heartburn.

Carcinoma of the oesophagus

This is a highly lethal disease. There are few reports of patients surviving for 5 years after diagnosis.

The disease is commoner in men than in women, and occurs particularly in old age. Predisposing factors include sideropenic dysphagia, achalasia and chronic oesophageal strictures, especially those resulting from the ingestion of corrosives. The bias towards females with sideropenic dysphagia explains why postcricoid carcinoma is more common in women than in men.

The histology of the tumour is usually epitheliomatous, arising from the squamous-celled epithelium of most of the oesophagus. However, at the lower end adenocarcinomas occur, arising from the glandular epithelium of the cardia which transgresses the anatomical boundary between oesophagus and stomach to a variable extent upwards. The lesion spreads by local extension, both up and down the gullet in the submucosal plane (where it may not be apparent to naked eye examination) and outwards to neighbouring structures such as the pericardium and heart, the carina of the oesophagus and roots of the lungs; and via the lymphatics, particularly with the left gastric artery to glands in the region of the coeliac artery, and upwards to the supraclavicular glands in the neck. The dissemination at an early stage, both locally to vital structures and to widespread regions, ensures that cure is unlikely.

Treatment

For the reasons given above, treatment has to be considered palliative. The main, and often only, symptom requiring palliation is dysphagia. Note that a gastrostomy is not worthwhile palliation because it does not enable the patient to swallow his own spittle.

The modalities of treatment available are surgery (bypass procedures, or extirpation with reconstruction of the food-tube), dilatation and intubation, and radiotherapy. Although radiotherapy is valueless for the adenocarcinoma of the lower end, it is the first line of treatment for the postcricoid lesions; if the latter have been detected at an early stage, they again form an exception to the general picture of oesophageal cancer in having an appreciable cure rate. Elsewhere in the oesophagus a combination of intubation to hold the lumen open plus radiotherapy to halt the growth of the lesion often gives effective palliation for many months. Tumours at the lower end of the oesophagus, particularly if they are adenocarcinomas, are often treated by oesophagogastrectomy via a thoracoabdominal approach. The left side of the thorax is opened in continuity with an upper abdominal incision, and the lower oesophagus excised with the whole, or upper half of the stomach (Fig. 2.5a). Reconstruction is by oesophagogastric or (Fig. 2.5d) oesophagojejunal anastomosis. A similar operation (the Ivor Lewis procedure) is also available for removing most of the thoracic oesophagus for tumours above the aortic arch: it involves separate incisions in the epigastrium and the right side of the chest (Fig. 2.5b). However, the mortality with these procedures is of the order of 20 per cent, mainly because of the tendency for the anastomosis to leak and the lethal effects of such a leak within the chest and mediastinum. There is an

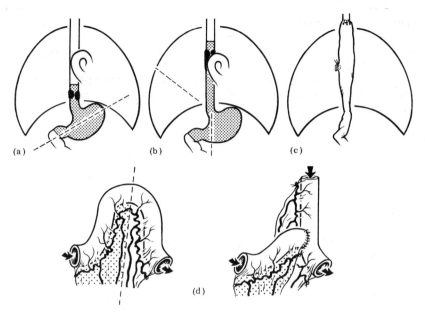

Fig. 2.5 Operations for carcinoma of the oesophagus. The shaded areas in (a) and (b) indicate the extent of the excision, and dotted lines the incisions. (a) Carcinoma of the lower third: abdominothoracic incision. The arch of the aorta prevents the surgeon from reaching the mid- or upper oesophagus by this route. (b) Carcinoma of the mid-oesophagus. Two separate incisions are used. Via the abdominal incision the stomach is mobilized and divided, either as indicated here at the duodenum if there is a suggestion of spread of the lesion into the stomach, or near its upper end. Via a right thoracotomy incision the oesophagus is mobilized to a level well above the tumour, and excised with the mobilized stomach. (c) It is possible to mobilize the stomach sufficiently to reach the neck for an anastomosis with the cervical oesophagus. This can be done leaving the oesophagus with its carcinoma *in situ* as palliation for irremovable growths, or after excision of the whole oesophagus via 'blind' cervical and abdominal approaches. (d) Principles for constructing a Roux-en-Y loop of jejunum for anastomosing with the cut end of the oesophagus. The mesentery of the proximal limb is shaded to aid its identification in the right hand of the two figures.

increasing move therefore to avoid anastomoses in the chest and either to excise the whole thoracic oesophagus or to bypass it, in both cases mobilizing stomach òr colon to bring it upwards via a tunnel in the mediastinum to an anastomosis with the cervical oesophagus (Fig. 2.5c).

Further reading

Earlam, R. J. (1975). *Clinical Tests of Oesophageal Function*. Crosby, Lockwood and Staples, London.

Editorial (1969). The Paterson–Kelly lesions. *British Medical Journal* **2**, 530.

Le Quesne, L. P. and Ranger, D. (1966). Pharyngolaryngectomy with immediate pharyngogastric anastomosis. *British Journal of Surgery* **53**, 105–109.

McKeown, K. C. (1972). Trends in oesophageal resection for carcinoma. *Annals of the Royal College of Surgeons of England* **51**, 213–239.

Smith, B. (1970). The neurological lesion in achalasia of the cardia. **Gut 11**, 388–391.

Vantrappen, G., Hellemans, J., Deloof, W., Valembois, P. and Vandenbroucke, J. (1971). Treatment of achalasia with pneumatic dilatations. *Gut* **12**, 268–275.

3

Upper abdominal symptoms

Patients with upper abdominal symptoms constitute the second-largest group (after the irritable colon syndrome) of all referrals to a medical gastroenterologist. The cardinal symptom is pain, which is usually epigastric or in the right quadrant but occasionally in the left, and usually has some temporal relationship with eating. Other symptoms include: *anorexia* or loss of appetite, *nausea, vomiting; heartburn*, a burning sensation in the lower substernal region, *waterbrash* and *bile regurgitation*, the regurgitation of, respectively, acid colourless or bitter yellow liquid into the mouth; and eructation, the upward expulsion of gas from the stomach—i.e. belching. Rarer complaints include abdominal distension, audible epigastric splash and symptoms referable to anaemia.

One or a combination of more than one of these symptoms is often described by the patient as 'indigestion', but since this term has no precise meaning it is better avoided completely. With sufficient encouragement, the patient is usually able to describe his symptoms in the precise terms of the previous paragraph. Particular care must be taken if the patient's description is colourful: the complaint of 'acid' or 'too much acid' may result from his projection that there is a known relation between gastric acid secretion and peptic ulceration, but the term may lead the unwary clinician to assume that his complaint is waterbrash when it may be something quite different.

Such symptoms are so common that every adult must surely have experienced them. In most cases the episode is brief and the frequency of further attacks low, so that the patient rarely seeks a medical opinion. Should the general practitioner be consulted, his past experience will enable him to reassure the majority that nothing serious is amiss, and a symptomatic remedy—usually in the form of an antacid preparation—is the only treatment necessary.

The problem is that upper abdominal symptoms *may* result from a serious disease of the oesophagus, stomach, duodenum or pancreaticobiliary apparatus. How does the practitioner select patients for referral to a gastro-enterologist at hospital? Some patients select themselves by making recurrent and frequent visits or by requesting a second opinion. Others alert the practitioner with evidence, from the history or examination, that is suggestive of serious disease.

The common conditions producing upper abdominal symptoms that require a specialist opinion are peptic ulcer, gallstones and reflux oesophagitis. Less common, but even more important because of their grave prognosis, are carcinoma of the stomach, carcinoma of the pancreas and chronic pancreatitis.

Peptic ulcer

Pathology

Peptic ulceration occurs only in the presence of acid–pepsin secretion from gastric mucosa, of which the parietal cells secrete a liquid containing hydrochloric acid and the chief cells secrete pepsin. Parietal and chief cells occur in the body and fundus of the stomach but not in the antrum. Heterotopic gastric mucosa is occasionally found; for example, at the lower end of the oesophagus, or even further afield in a Meckel's diverticulum.

The nature of the relationship between acid–pepsin secretion by the stomach and peptic ulceration, and other factors known or suspected to be of aetiological importance, are described in Chapter 4.

Traditionally, there are two forms of peptic ulcer—*acute* and *chronic*—but the distinction is often difficult. The acute ulcer is often (but not always—it can be as deep as a chronic ulcer) a shallow erosion of the mucosa, found anywhere in the stomach or first part of the duodenum, usually producing no symptoms unless it causes haemorrhage, and is associated with stress (Chapter 7). The chronic ulcer has perpendicular walls ('punched out') and is much deeper. It always extends through the muscularis mucosae and often through the whole muscular wall and serous covering of the stomach so that its floor is the tissue of a neighbouring viscus, often the pancreas. The site of chronic peptic ulcers is characteristic: they occur where non-acid-secreting mucosa is exposed to acid–pepsin—i.e. at the margin of areas containing parietal and chief cells. This statement applies to the rare oesophageal or Meckel's diverticulum ulcer, and to the stomach itself where gastric ulcers are found at or near the lesser curvature, just on the antral side of the demarcation between acid-secreting and antral mucosa. Gastric ulcers often occur much higher on the lesser curve than on the incisura which is the traditional site for the corpus/antrum junction, but in such patients it is always found that there is a tongue of antral mucosa extending proximally along the lesser curvature to the site of the ulcer. The duodenal ulcer is an apparent exception to the general statement, but even this lesion occurs usually in the most proximal part of the duodenum, at the junction between pyloric and duodenal mucosa, and not far from the acid-secreting mucosa.

The chronic peptic ulcer which produces upper abdominal symptoms is discussed in this chapter. Acute ulcers, and the acute complications of chronic ulcers—bleeding, perforation and obstruction—are considered in Chapter 7.

Carcinoma of the duodenum is very rare, and therefore a duodenal ulcer, once diagnosed, can be confidently accepted to be benign. The same is not true of gastric ulcers: the diagnosis of such an ulcer should always raise the possibility in the mind of the clinician that it may represent, from the outset, a carcinoma of the stomach (p. 38); a small percentage of peptic ulcers of the stomach, perhaps 1–5 per cent, show a tendency to malignant change.

History

The cardinal feature is *pain*, which is usually midline epigastric in site but may be substernal or in the right upper quadrant. The pain seems to be related to emptiness of the stomach because it is relieved by food, returning ½–2 hours after the previous meal—presumably when gastric emptying is complete—never starting during a meal, and often waking the patient in the small hours of the morning. The link between the pain and the production of hydrochloric acid by the stomach is emphasized by the fact that alkaline liquids such as milk and alkaline pharmaceutical preparations (antacids) are particularly effective in relieving the pain.

The pain is typically described as dull or burning, and it may radiate through to the back, a feature which suggests *penetration* by the ulcer through the whole thickness of the stomach wall into the pancreas because pain from the pancreas is usually referred to the back.

The single feature of a pain which most suggests that it originates in a peptic ulcer is that it is neither continuous nor sporadic but periodic. The patient does not have pain every day for months on end, nor a severe attack on 1 day only and then no more pain for months; rather, he has pain every day after most meals for 2 or 3 weeks, then a period of complete remission lasting for several weeks or months, and then another bout starts.

Symptoms other than pain are more variable, less specific and correspondingly more difficult to assess. The patient may complain of *weight loss* resulting from being afraid to eat because he knows that shortly after the meal he will get his pain, or of *weight gain* due to drinking an excess of milk in order to relieve the pain. *Heartburn* and *eructations* are ascribed to spasm of the pylorus with an increase in pressure that results in the reflux of acid and gas into the lower oesophagus but this explanation, though convincing, is unproven. *Nausea* and *vomiting* may accompany the pain and are perhaps also due to pyloric spasm; vomiting usually relieves the pain, and the vomitus is characteristically small in volume and consists of liquid, mostly bile. This last feature suggests that the zone of high pressure is in the duodenum rather than at the pylorus.

Signs

There are few physical signs with an uncomplicated peptic ulcer. The most common is epigastric tenderness, but even this is not usually apparent. Obesity or evidence of weight loss may be noted, and there is said to be a characteristic facies in older males: a lean, haggard face with deeply furrowed nasolabial grooves. A suggestive history alone should lead to special investigations (p. 25).

Gallstones

The precipitation of various chemical substances normally held in soluble form in the bile and the consequent formation of calculi is a process which, apart from exceptional (p. 22) circumstances, occurs only in the gall bladder.

Stones are commonly encountered in other parts of the biliary passages but they have arisen in the gall bladder and this fact has a strong influence on treatment.

Pathology

There are two principal chemical varieties: the *pigment stone* and the *cholesterol stone*. In both types, but especially the latter, a variable quantity of calcium salts may become incorporated in the stones, particularly in their outer layers because the process is at least partially physical adsorption, and there is a resultant increase in opacity to x-rays (p. 28).

Pigment stones result from the excessive haemolysis of erythrocytes in haemolytic anaemias (p. 78); the pigment is bilirubin and related products. These stones are always multiple and characteristically small. *Cholesterol stones* result from a failure of the normal mechanisms that keep this insoluble product of metabolism in a form of solution in bile (Sanford: *Digestive System Physiology*, Chapter 4); they may be solitary and spherical (the 'cholesterol solitaire'), or multiple and facetted.

The wall of a gall bladder containing stones of either type may be histologically normal. This suggests that the major factor confining stone formation to this organ rather than allowing it to take place in other parts of the biliary passages is some normal function of the gall bladder. One might expect this function to be *concentration*: gall bladder bile is several times more concentrated than common bile duct bile in most of its constituents, including cholesterol. The concentration effect results from absorption of electrolytes and, subsequently, water (Sanford: *Digestive System Physiology*, Chapter 4). However, the true reason seems to be the stasis factor which is always present in the gall bladder as distinct from the rest of the biliary tract. This fact explains why, once a gall bladder containing stones has been surgically removed, and provided that there is no abnormality present in the bile ducts, no new stones form in the ducts even though nothing has been done to reduce the original metabolic factor. Stone formation *can* take place in the bile ducts, but only in the presence of a foreign body to act as a nucleus for precipitation. The most commonly occurring foreign body is a gallstone which has been produced in the gall bladder but migrated into the duct. It is therefore most important that the surgeon removing the gall bladder containing stones checks whether there are any stones in the bile ducts and removes such stones as well. In South-east Asia there is another cause of intraductal formation of calculi—the liver fluke, *Clonorchis sinensis*.

Gallstones, like foreign bodies anywhere else in the tissues, predispose to infection and so the wall of the gall bladder may show the changes of chronic inflammation. Prominent among the histological features of chronic cholecystitis are Rokitansky–Aschoff sinuses, which are probably pulsion diverticula into the submucosa—certainly they sometimes rupture with extravasation of bile into the tissues of the wall of the gall bladder.

The most important complication of gallstones lying within the gall bladder is acute cholecystitis. A gallstone impacts in the neck of the viscus where Hartmann's pouch joins the cystic duct. Pressure rises within the organ as mucus secretion into its lumen continues. A severe mechanical inflammation of the gall bladder ensues. This is in most cases eventually relieved by the disimpaction of the stone, but occasionally secondary infection by the organisms inseparable from any foreign body may first occur. Thus in acute cholecystitis spontaneous resolution is the rule, but rupture of the organ if the pressure within it markedly rises or complications such as septicaemia if secondary infection occurs are not unknown.

Acute cholecystitis occasionally occurs in the absence of gallstones. The aetiology is unknown.

Other complications of gallstones include obstructive jaundice (p. 80) or ascending cholangitis (p. 83) due to stones that have migrated from the gall bladder into the common bile duct via the cystic duct, or (rarely) *gallstone ileus*, mechanical obstruction of the ileum near its termination (where the lumen of the bowel is narrowest) by a gallstone. A stone large enough to impact at this point is too large to have passed along the cystic duct, and has probably entered the duodenum by eroding through the contiguous walls of the gall bladder and the duodenum, i.e. via a cholecystoduodenal fistula.

Gallstones are very common in the Western world, and cholecystectomy is probably the second most common major operation in Europe and North America (after vascular bypass procedures for coronary artery disease). Stones are frequently found at post-mortem examination in subjects who had had no abdominal complaints during life. In developing countries they are at present rare, but as the standard of living in such countries rises, and particularly as the diet changes from traditional to Western pattern, the incidence of gallstones increases dramatically. Women are affected more commonly than men, and the peak incidence is around 45 years of age although the disease is becoming more common in younger patients; the reasons for this change remain obscure.

History

The standard teaching has been that gallstones are associated with *flatulent dyspepsia*; that is, some combination of upper abdominal symptoms in which distension and eructations are prominent, and that these symptoms are worse with fatty foods. The truth seems to be that fat intolerance is a rare condition—the complaint that a patient cannot eat fatty food is usually no more than a food fad—and that flatulent dyspepsia and gallstones are both common phenomena and therefore by coincidence are frequently encountered in the same subject. It is probable that stones lying within the gall bladder produce no symptoms unless complications arise.

A history suggestive of gallstones is thus a history suggestive of the common complication, impaction of a stone in the neck of the gall bladder. The patient complains of one or more attacks of severe upper abdominal pain, requiring opiates for its relief. Each attack beings gradually, builds up to its maximal level, and lasts for several hours or even 2 or 3 days. The pain is epigastric or in the right upper quadrant of the abdomen, and it radiates through the body, or round the lower right ribs, to the back. Occasionally there is the classic radiation to the right shoulder-tip of pain resulting from diaphragmatic irritation, conveyed via the phrenic and supraclavicular nerves, both of which are derived from the third to fifth cervical nerve roots. The pain is often described as gripping, and the time-relations of the attacks, their long duration without respite and their sporadic distribution without any recognizable pattern are in sharp contrast to the symptoms of peptic ulceration.

Jaundice may occur during an attack: the patient's sclerae become yellow, and since the jaundice is obstructive in nature the stools become pale ('putty-coloured') and the urine dark (p. 80). The obstruction can be due to the presence of a stone in the common duct, but there seems to be no doubt that jaundice can occur in the absence of a stone in the common duct and must therefore presumably be due to a functional disturbance of the drainage of bile along the duct, perhaps resulting from oedema and acute inflammation.

Signs

At the usual time when the patient is seen (that is, between acute attacks when he is symptomless), there are no abnormal physical signs apart from the obesity that is so common in patients with gallstones. Occasionally, Murphy's sign is positive: the examiner's hand palpating deeply in the right hypochondrium elicits pain at the extreme of deep inspiration. For the findings during an acute attack, see p. 112.

Reflux oesophagitis

Pathology

Reflux oesophagitis is a condition in which inflammation of a variable length of the lower oesophagus occurs as a combination of areas of acute inflammation superimposed on a wider background of chronic inflammation. The worst changes are at the lower end, but the process can extend upwards to the level of the arch of the aorta or beyond.

This condition seems to be associated with reflux of acid–pepsin from the stomach into the lower oesophagus, and there is evidence that the inflammation is aggravated by the presence of bile in the reflux, patients with the worst oesophagitis tending to have the highest concentrations of bile salts in fasting gastric juice.

Gastro-oesophageal reflux is common. Its incidence probably increases with age: over the age of 50 years a prevalence approaching 1 in 3 is often quoted. Reflux commonly coexists with a sliding hiatus hernia (p. 30), but not all patients with a hernia have reflux nor do all patients with reflux have a hernia.

The inflammatory process tends to destroy the mucosa, producing ulceration. The reparative powers of the mucosa must be excellent because it is not unusual to find inflammatory changes in the biopsy specimen of a region of submucosa despite an overlying area of apparently normal mucosa. When regeneration is finally outstripped, a raw bleeding area of submucosa is left exposed and iron-deficiency anaemia is a recognized sequel. Healing takes place by fibrosis with contracture and consequent stricture formation. A rare complication of long-standing chronic ulceration and fibrosis is malignant change, i.e. carcinoma of the lower oesophagus.

History

The cardinal complaint of patients with oesophagitis is heartburn. The symptom occurs particularly when the pressure within the stomach is high, either because the organ is full and actively secreting acid–pepsin during or shortly after a meal, or because the intra-abdominal pressure is high. The most important causes of raised intra-abdominal pressure (relative to the intraoesophageal or intrathoracic pressure) are pregnancy, posture and obesity; the symptom is exacerbated by lying down, stooping, or, on a more extended time-scale, by putting on weight.

Symptoms in long-standing cases include those of chronic anaemia (malaise, tiredness, dyspnoea on effort) and dysphagia due to a stricture (p. 31).

Signs

There are no abnormal signs specifically suggesting this condition.

First-line investigations

A clinical picture suggesting that the patient may have organic disease in the upper abdomen leads to a cholecystogram, barium meal or both. These may be thought of as first-line investigations in the sense that they are available at all major hospitals, they are well established procedures, and the methods of performance and interpretation of the results are standard. If the clinician thinks that the odds favour disease of the gall bladder rather than of the oesophagus, stomach and duodenum, or *vice versa*, then the appropriate investigation is requested first. If the odds seem equally balanced, the cholecystogram is usually performed first since the contrast material used in that investigation disappears more rapidly from the upper abdomen than the barium salt used in a barium meal examination and there is thus less chance of the first investigation interfering with the interpretation of the second. The three diseases concerned are so common that it is not unusual for two of them, or even all three, to coexist; it has therefore been suggested that *both* investigations should always be done as a routine, but this is a counsel of perfection that would be expensive to implement.

Barium meal (upper gastrointestinal opaque meal)

The patient drinks a suspension of an insoluble barium salt, and the radiologist observes the gullet, stomach and duodenal region on the fluoroscopic screen and takes still films at appropriate moments. With the first few swallows, the passage of the meal along the oesophagus is traced and any abnormality noted. Peptic oesophagitis as such produces no diagnostic appearances, but a stricture shows as a smooth narrowing of the lower end of the gullet. The smoothness is in contradistinction to the ragged appearance and 'shoulders' of a carcinoma of the lower oesophagus (see Fig. 2.3b), but these features cannot be relied upon as evidence that there is no cancer present. Only biopsy, if necessary repeated, can establish that. (For other abnormal appearances in these early stages of the meal, usually referred to as the barium swallow, see p. 12.)

When more of the meal has been swallowed the stomach becomes outlined. A benign (peptic) gastric ulcer of the chronic variety (acute erosions are rarely visualized by a barium meal) presents as an outpouching (the ulcer niche) from the stomach wall, nearly always somewhere along the lesser curvature (Fig. 3.1). A site removed from the lesser curvature, or any suggestion that the ulcer crater lies on a mass projecting into the lumen of the stomach, is a feature pointing strongly towards a diagnosis of carcinoma of the stomach. A double-contrast technique using air as well as barium increases accuracy.

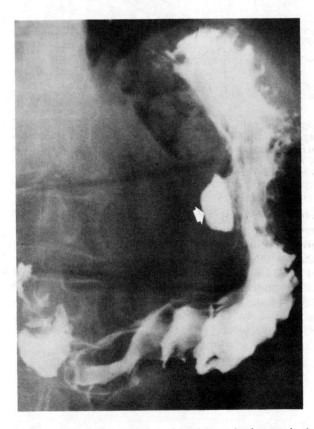

Fig. 3.1 Barium meal showing a niche due to a benign gastric ulcer at the typical site on the lesser curve (arrow).

The competence of the cardiac sphincter and the possibility that a hiatal hernia is present are investigated by raising the intragastric pressure. The patient is tilted so that his feet are higher than his head, and compression applied to the abdomen by an abdominal binder. The appearances of gastro-oesophageal reflux and of the sliding type of hiatal hernia (Fig. 3.2a) usually coexist (p. 24), but the rarer paraoesophageal hernia or rolling type (Fig. 3.2b) in which the cardia stays below the diaphragm and a pouch of greater curvature protrudes from the abdomen alongside the oesophagus in a peritoneal sac may also be demonstrated.

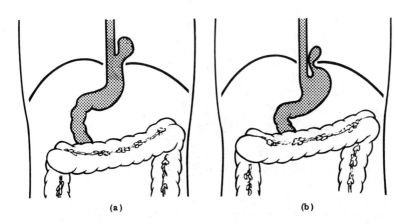

(a)   (b)

Fig. 3.2 Hiatal hernia: the two main types. (a) Sliding: the cardio-oesophageal junction lies above the diaphragm. (b) Paraoesophageal or rolling: the cardio-oesophageal junction stays below the diaphragm and a pouch of greater curvature herniates through the diaphragm beside the oesophagus. A mixed type, combining the features of both, also occurs.

Finally, the duodenum is closely inspected. Radiologists call the first part of the duodenum the duodenal cap, and a normal one is a capacious structure (Fig. 3.3). This appearance is not seen all the time because the gross anatomy of the region is often distorted by peristalsis, but it should be demonstrable in at least one film out of the several taken of this area. The typical radiological feature of most cases of duodenal ulcer is *persistent* distortion of the cap, which is never seen in the relaxed condition; occasionally, with careful positioning of the patient, an ulcer crater with folds of mucous membrane radiating from it can be demonstrated. The radiological diagnosis of a duodenal ulcer is usually less precise than that of a gastric ulcer.

Cholecystography

The standard technique for opacifying the gall bladder is the *oral cholecystogram*. The patient swallows an organic iodide (iopanoic acid, Telepaque) which is absorbed from the gastrointestinal tract and excreted by the liver in the bile. The concentration in the hepatic bile is not usually high enough to show the

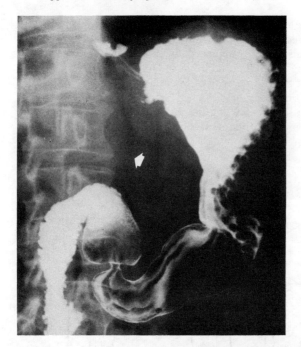

Fig. 3.3 Barium meal showing a normal duodenal cap (arrow). If the cap fails to show this typical voluminous shape in *any* of the views, it is likely that a duodenal ulcer (or a healed ulcer) is present.

common bile duct, but after further concentration in the gall bladder the gall bladder itself becomes visible.

Gallstones containing sufficient calcium may be seen on the preliminary plain film of the gall bladder region (Fig. 3.4a), and their nature confirmed by their appearance as filling defects in the opacified gall bladder (Fig. 3.4b).

If the gall bladder does not opacify (the so-called non-functioning gall bladder), the possible causes are that the patient has not taken the contrast, that the material has not been absorbed, that it has not been concentrated adequately by the liver or that it cannot get into the gall bladder because the cystic duct is blocked. In such patients a different examination, an *intravenous cholangiogram*, is performed. A different organic iodide that is water-soluble is injected intravenously, and the concentration achieved in the hepatic bile is adequate to outline the bile ducts. If, despite adequate visualization of the common bile duct, the gall bladder is still not seen then the cystic duct must be blocked. The cause is almost always a stone impacted in the duct (or in Hartmann's pouch).

For the role of ultrasonography in the investigation of the biliary tract, see p. 38.

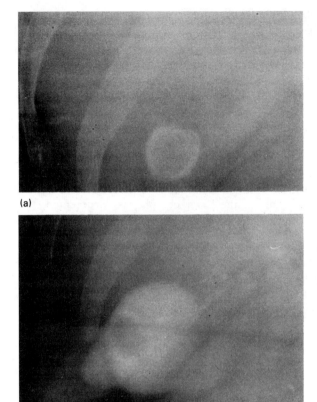

(a)

(b)

Fig. 3.4 (a) Plain x-ray of the right upper quadrant of the abdomen, showing gallstone. (b) Cholecystogram. The opacification of the gall bladder confirms the presence of the stone as a filling defect.

Further management

After the first-line investigations the patient is reassessed with the results. Sometimes a precise diagnosis of one of the three common conditions has been achieved. The management of gallstones and of gastro-oesophageal reflux is described below, and that of peptic ulcer in Chapter 4. Rarer conditions identified are dealt with on their merits.

Sometimes the radiological appearances are entirely normal. The clinician must decide whether to reassure the patient or whether to embark on more complicated investigations. Relevant considerations include the duration of the history, the persistence of the symptoms, the patient's attitude towards them, the experience of the clinician and the presence of certain features that suggest one of the less common but more serious diseases—carcinoma of the stomach, carcinoma of the pancreas or chronic pancreatitis.

Gastro-oesophageal reflux/hiatal hernia

The radiological demonstration of reflux or of a hiatal hernia (often both) makes it likely that the heartburn related to posture, or less characteristic symptoms, is due to reflux oesophagitis. It is important to exclude the possibility that the radiological abnormalities are coincidental, because these abnormalities are very common and can undoubtedly be symptomless. Therefore, endoscopy is always performed. The lower end of the oesophagus is inspected, the zone of inflammation noted and its extent measured, the presence of gastric juice or bile in the lower oesophagus documented, the distance from the incisor teeth at which gastric epithelium starts (normally 40 cm) measured, any stricture calibrated in relation to the size of the endoscope, and biopsies taken. The biopsies are particularly important if a stricture is present because it might be due to carcinoma, and in puzzling cases apparently without oesophagitis where the inflammatory changes are found deep to a normal-looking mucosa.

Treatment

The aim is to avoid the reflux of gastric contents into the lower oesophagus, and if that is not possible to protect the mucosa of the oesophagus from their effects.

The most important advice to give a patient who is overweight, even if only moderately, is to lose weight. The effect of weight loss on symptoms can be dramatic. Other measures to reduce intragastric pressure include the avoidance of tight garments and of acts involving bending and stooping; meals should be kept small in bulk and alcohol and tobacco reduced or eliminated. At night the patient is usually much less troubled by heartburn if the head of his bed is raised on 25 cm (10 inch) blocks. Antacids are prescribed to be taken after meals and for the relief of symptoms at other times (they should be kept by the bedside at night), and they are particularly effective if they are combined with a surface-forming agent such as methylcellulose. Cimetidine to reduce the ability of the stomach to secrete acid also has its advocates.

Such measures are usually effective, and even an early stricture might resolve. Occasionally the symptoms continue, and justify a surgical attempt to prevent reflux. Until recently the focus of surgical attack has been on the sliding hiatal hernia that is usually present. Competence at the cardia seems to be related to an intrinsic zone of high pressure in the lower 1 or 2 cm of the oesophagus, despite the absence of any anatomically identifiable sphincter at that site (Sanford: *Disgestive System Physiology*, Chapter 1), and it has been assumed that exposure of this region to the lower intrathoracic pressure, when the cardia slides above the diaphragm, rather than to the higher intra-abdominal pressure is the main factor producing incontinence that must be corrected. Many different operations to repair a sliding hiatal hernia have therefore been described, and their very number illustrates that none is very successful in keeping the stomach below the diaphragm. The difficulty is to maintain approximation of the crura tightly enough around the lower oesophagus to prevent the stomach slipping upwards: stitches tend to cut out. Recently a much more successful approach has been devised: the fundus of the stomach is mobilized, wrapped round the lower end of oesophagus and fixed in that position (Fig. 3.5). This manoeuvre results in the lower oesophagus always being subjected to the higher intragastric (i.e. intra-abdominal) pressure, even if it has slid up into the chest.

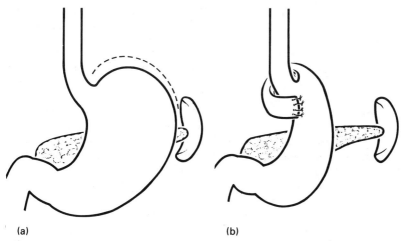

(a)   (b)

Fig. 3.5 The wrap-round operation for prevention of gastro-oesophageal reflux (Nissen procedure). (a) The greater curvature is mobilized as far as necessary by division of the short gastric vessels running in the greater omentum between the stomach and the upper pole of the spleen. (b) The mobilized fundus is wrapped round the lower oesophagus and fixed anteriorly.

An established stricture of the lower oesophagus due to peptic oesophagitis is a very difficult condition to treat. *Once a stricture, always a stricture* is an old surgical maxim which is fortunately not so accurate here as elsewhere. Repeated dilatation of the lower oesophagus under endoscopic control relieves the dysphagia; the procedure usually has to be repeated, but by no means necessarily indefinitely. The risk of accidental perforation of the oesophagus, with the consequent features of mediastinitis—severe pain, profound collapse and pyrexia—and a high mortality rate, increases proportionately. A combination of dilatation to a full calibre followed by a good anti-reflux operation sometimes works, but excision of the stricture and reanastomosis to the stomach is sometimes necessary. The trouble is that this operation itself destroys the cardia, and so the scene is set for more reflux.

Gallstones

The presence of one or more calculi within the gall bladder is an indication for *cholecystectomy*, the operation of removing the gall bladder. This statement requires two qualifications: first, in a patient without severe symptoms from his gallstones and whose medical condition in other respects makes him a bad surgical risk, it is reasonable to defer operation in the hope that no uncomfortable or dangerous complications of the gallstones arise; secondly, the possibility of dissolving gallstones by chemical methods is now real and is discussed below. Nevertheless, the main statement that gallstones are an indication for cholecystectomy remains true; several centres have reported that patients with gallstones in whom the diagnosis was made coincidentally—for example, on a chest x-ray—and who have no symptoms referable to their gallstones, have a high incidence of the complications of gallstones during a 5-year period of follow-up. Because the complications are life-threatening, and increase the morbidity and mortality of operative treatment, the consensus of opinion is that gallstones, even when symptomless, should be removed. Note that the gall bladder as well as the stones must be removed (p. 83).

Cholecystectomy

This operation can be technically easy, or one of the most difficult in the abdomen. The steps are to identify and divide the cystic artery and the cystic duct, the latter at its junction with the common hepatic and common bile ducts; the gall bladder can then be peeled off its hepatic bed, working from neck to fundus. Technical problems are due either to inflammatory or post-inflammatory changes (oedema, injection, adhesions) which obscure the features of the anatomy, or to variations of anatomy that are common in this region and might lead the unwary surgeon to cut the right hepatic artery instead of the cystic or a common duct instead of the cystic duct. The operation is performed through an upper abdominal oblique, transverse or vertical incision, and on average the patient is in hospital between 7 and 10 days.

Stones in the common ducts (choledocholithiasis)

Another major problem during cholecystectomy is the possibility that stones have already migrated from the gall bladder into the common duct. Because such stones can produce obstructive jaundice by impaction at the lower end of the common bile duct or predispose to infection (cholangitis), both conditions that gravely threaten life, common duct stones should be removed during the operation. On the other hand, exploring the common bile duct has been shown to lead to a longer average duration of stay in hospital, and probably also to increased morbidity and even mortality compared with cholecystectomy alone. Exploration can, for example, introduce infection (cholangitis), or produce traumatic oedema and spasm at the lower end of the common bile duct, thereby interfering with drainage down the pancreatic duct and causing acute pancreatitis (p. 108).

To reduce the number of unnecessary explorations of the common duct, the standard technique is *preoperative cholangiography*. After the cystic duct has been exposed it is cannulated, and a radio-opaque contrast medium (e.g. 25 per cent diodone) injected. If the criteria of a normal common duct system are met

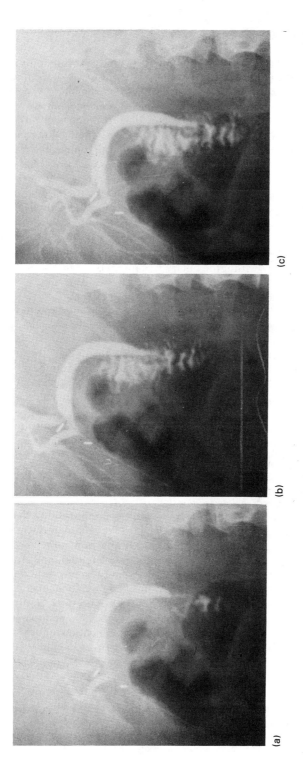

(a)

(b)

(c)

Fig. 3.6 The radiographic criteria of a normal cholangiogram. The common bile duct contains no filling defects and does not exceed 12 mm. in diameter; there is free flow of contrast medium into the duodenum in at least the second and third films, the narrow terminal segment is seen on at least one film, and there is not obvious distension of the hepatic duct radicles.

(Fig. 3.6), there is no need to explore the duct. If this radiographic technique is not available, the surgeon perforce relies on the much less accurate clinical indications for exploration: a recent history of jaundice, the presence of several small stones in the gall bladder and palpability of stones within the duct.

If exploration is decided upon, the common bile duct is opened (choledochotomy) through a 1 cm incision below the entrance of the cystic duct, and special instruments (Desjardin's forceps) are passed up and down the biliary passages. After any stones present have been removed, the patency of the lower end of the duct is checked by passing a soft plastic bougie down through the duct into the duodenum. A flexible choledochoscope is now available, and some surgeons use it routinely to view the inside of the ducts. The hole in the common duct is sewn up round a T-tube drain (Fig. 3.7) because spasm of the sphincter of Oddi is common after exploration and the resultant high pressure within the biliary tree might burst the suture line in the duct were the T-tube not there to act as a safety-valve. A postexploratory cholangiogram can be performed on the operating-table, although spasm and the difficulty of eliminating air-bubbles make its interpretation more equivocal than that of the pre-exploratory films. Ten days after the operation,

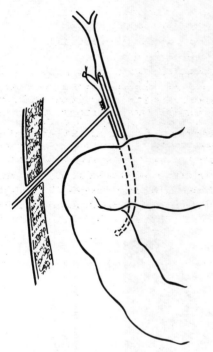

Fig. 3.7   The principle of T-tube drainage after choledochotomy. The short limb of the T-tube is usually guttered rather than cylindrical, to reduce the risk of blockage. Any interference with the drainage of bile into the duodenum results in flow out along the long limb through the abdominal wall to be collected in a drainage bag, and prevents any back-pressure within the common duct that might rupture the sutured incision in its wall.

more cholangiographic films are obtained via the T-tube; if these show no evidence of stones and confirm that there is free drainage into the duodenum, the T-tube is removed. The resulting fistula leaks a few millilitres of bile but has usually healed within 2 or 3 days.

Retained common duct stones
Despite all precautions during cholecystectomy, the problem of stones left in the common duct is not uncommon (Fig. 3.8).

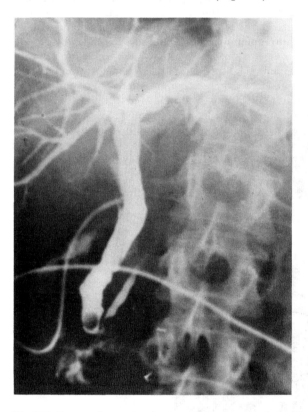

Fig. 3.8 Peroperative postexploratory cholangiogram via the T-tube, showing a moderately dilated common bile duct with a filling defect due to a residual stone near the lower end. The surgeon had thought he had cleared the common duct of all stones, and the value of the postexploratory film is obvious.

The patient presents with attacks suggestive of acute cholecystitis, or with obstructive jaundice, or with the rigors and prostration of ascending cholangitis. After the attack has subsided, an intravenous cholangiogram (there is no point in trying oral cholangiography after cholecystectomy, p. 28) may demonstrate a dilated common bile duct, perhaps with filling defects.

Until recently the only form of treatment available was surgical; i.e. an operation to explore the bile ducts and remove the stones. Technically such a procedure after previous cholecystectomy can be very difficult, and it is fortunate that another mode of management is now available. A flexible gastroduodenoscope is passed via the mouth into the second part of the duodenum. A channel within this apparatus is used first to cannulate the papilla of Vater so as to obtain accurate cholangiographic evidence of the number and size of the stones; next to slit the orifice with a diathermy electrode so that the stones are more likely to pass spontaneously into the duodenum; and even to pass up the duct instruments capable of snaring a stone so that withdrawal of the instrument removes the stone (Fig. 3.9). The minority of stones that are too large or too firmly impacted to be amenable to endoscopic techniques require open operation.

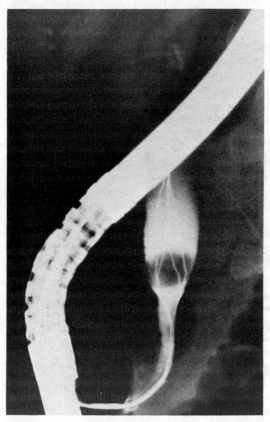

Fig. 3.9 Removal of stones from common bile duct with a wire basket introduced via a duodenoscope.

Dissolution of gallstones
Cholesterol is insoluble in water, and the cholesterol excreted in the bile by the liver is only kept in solution in the form of micelles with bile acids and lecithin (Sanford: *Digestive System Physiology*, Chapter 4). Patients with cholesterol gallstones have been shown to excrete in hepatic bile a larger concentration of

cholesterol than normal subjects so that hepatic bile is superconcentrated for cholesterol. Despite this superconcentration, the cholesterol does not precipitate until exposed to the effect of stasis in the gall bladder. Factors involved in the solubility of cholesterol thus include its rate of excretion from the liver and the availability of the bile salts.

It has been found that the ingestion of one of the primary bile acids, chenodeoxycholic acid (CDC), in a daily dose of 15 mg/kg body weight has the effect of dissolving cholesterol stones. It works probably through at least two effects—a reduction in the output and concentration of cholesterol in hepatic bile and an increase in the bile salt pool. Recently a similar substance isolated from bears, and called ursodeoxycholic acid, has been found to have similar effects.

The rate of dissolution is slow, and treatment has to continue for several months or years, during which time the patient is still at risk from complications. Large stones respond more slowly than average, calcified stones not at all. Most important of all, even when stones have been completely dissolved, if the treatment is stopped then recurrent stone formation is the almost universal rule. For this reason the medical treatment of gallstones is still a research tool rather than a practicable alternative to surgery—unless there are strong medical contraindications to operation.

Incidentally, some of the factors known to be associated with an increased incidence of gallstones have been shown to work via the mechanism described. The increasing incidence with age and in the female sex are unexplained, but the very high incidence in the American Pima Indians is probably due to an increased hepatic secretion of cholesterol and a reduced formation of bile salts. The nature of the association of cholesterol gallstones with carcinoma of the gall bladder is not clear, though the latter may result from the irritation of the wall of the gall bladder by long-standing gallstones. Disease or operative removal of the terminal ileum reduces the bile salt pool size, because it is in this region of the bowel that bile salts are normally reabsorbed to the extent of about 95 per cent. The irritant effect of bile salts on the large bowel is prominent in patients with intestinal hurry (p. 158), and if this condition is treated with cholestyramine, an agent that combines with bile salts, the incidence of gallstones subsequently is high. Vagotomy may have its effect through diminishing the ability of the gall bladder to empty itself, thus encouraging stasis. The normal stimulus to gall bladder contraction is the hormone cholecystokinin-pancreozymin (CCK-PZ), which is released from the duodenal mucosa in response to the presence of fat in the duodenum. This release of the hormone is partially dependent on an intact vagal innervation. The association of gallstones with acute pancreatitis is discussed elsewhere (p. 109).

Cholesterol stones are probably more common in obese patients, and there is no doubt that supersaturation of hepatic bile with cholesterol is more common in the obese although the linking mechanism is unknown. Finally, drugs used to lower the level of cholesterol in the blood in an attempt to prevent atheroma (e.g. clofibrate) are likely to produce gallstones. Thus the metabolism of fat is closely bound up with cholesterol stone formation in ways we do not yet understand.

Second-line investigations

If the first-line investigations have yielded normal results but the clinician thinks the likelihood of serious disease in a particular patient is high, or if the first-line investigations have suggested a lesion other than duodenal ulcer or gallstones, further investigations are requested. In addition to x-ray-negative peptic ulcer, the chief diseases to be considered are gastric cancer, chronic pancreatitis and cancer of the pancreas. Important clinical features suggesting the presence of serious disease include anorexia and weight loss, severe and unremitting pain, particularly with radiation through to the back, and steatorrhoea (p. 42). The onset of jaundice puts the problem into a separate category (Chapter 6).

The two principal modes of investigation are *ultrasonography* and *gastro-duodenoscopy*, the latter extended if necessary by the cannulation of bile and pancreatic ducts—endoscopic retrograde cholangio-pancreatography (ERCP). Ultrasonography is one of the most useful of the newer techniques in medical investigation. It is rapid, simple, non-invasive, relatively cheap and, in the present context, valuable for demonstrating a mass distorting the normal shape of the pancreas (i.e. a carcinoma of the pancreas). Since it can also demonstrate gallstones, distended bile ducts and a distended gall bladder with good reliability, some authorities would place this technique among the first-line investigations. Its drawback is that the interpretation of ultrasonograms requires skilled interpretation, and such skills are at present concentrated in special centres. They are diffusing rapidly, and the emphasis on ultrasonography is steadily increasing.

During the last two decades endoscopy has also made astonishing advances, principally because of the invention of fibreoptics, a process whereby light rays are bent round corners by internal reflections along a system of flexible glass cylinders, the fibres of the title. The flexibility of the resulting gastroscopes has transformed what was a dangerous (perforation of the oesophagus) procedure yielding a limited view into a safe operation, readily performed on outpatients under sedation, giving an unhurried and accurate view of oesophagus, stomach and duodenum, and affording the opportunity for the taking of biopsies and of brush-scrapings for cytological examination, and for cannulating the bile and pancreatic ducts. Many authorities consider endoscopy (without cannulation) to be a first-line investigation replacing the barium meal. There is no doubt, for example, that not all peptic ulcers are demonstrated by an opaque meal x-ray series, and endoscopy permits biopsy, a tremendous advantage over radiology. All gastric ulcers demonstrated by radiology, no matter how benign they appear (p. 26), should be biopsied because gastric carcinoma is quite common, and so it is argued that the endoscopy might as well be the first investigation. The army of skilled endoscopists is gradually growing, but the average situation world-wide at present is still that the barium meal is more readily available.

Carcinoma of the stomach

Cancer of the stomach rates third among the most common causes of death from malignant disease in the United Kingdom. The prognosis is grave: only 1 patient in 20 lives for 5 years after diagnosis in this country.

Aetiology

The incidence of gastric carcinoma is decreasing. While still very common in most parts of the world, and while the geographical variation in incidence is remarkably wide—the incidence in Japan is 30 times the incidence in Mozambique—this statement is true in every area for which adequate statistics are available. Moreover, Japanese immigrants in the United States have an incidence intermediate between native Americans and Japanese living in Japan, and there are studies showing a similar phenomenon in other immigrant groups. It appears, therefore, that the factors producing gastric carcinoma are predominantly environmental, although there is some evidence of a genetic predisposition: a slightly increased incidence among the relatives of patients and an association with blood group A.

The environmental factors concerned are undoubtedly multiple. Cigarette smoking definitely increases the risk whilst milk and fresh vegetables have a protective effect. Otherwise nothing has been proven to be an important factor, although there is increasing evidence that a high concentration of nitrates in food is harmful. The theory is that nitrates, after reduction to nitrites, react with amines to form nitrosamines, a class of compound known to be strongly carcinogenic in animal experiments. The link with smoking might be explained by the fact that there are high concentrations of thiocyanate—an ion which facilitates the formation of nitrosamines—in the saliva of smokers. There is also a reported link with smoked and pickled foods, the preserving processes for which involve nitrates.

Patients with the complete achlorhydria of pernicious anaemia (p. 53) have a definite risk of gastric carcinoma, and there is a statistical association between chronic atrophic gastritis (a condition producing hypochlorhydria) and gastric carcinoma. There is no doubt that some patients with cancer of the stomach secrete acid in normal quantities, but it is possible that atrophic gastritis is a local predisposing factor.

Pathology

The lesion is an adenocarcinoma, varying from the well differentiated or *intestinal* type predominating in older patients to the undifferentiated or *diffuse* type seen often in younger patients.

Spread is, at least at first, mainly to the neighbouring lymph nodes—along the main gastric arterial pedicles of the right and left gastroepiploic and right and left gastric arteries, and thence to nodes along the coeliac axis and the posterior abdominal wall around the aorta, along the splenic vessels in relation to the tail and body of the pancreas, and along the pancreaticoduodenal vessels to the head of the pancreas and the hepatic to the porta hepatis. Thus very rapidly there is spread by the lymphatics to a variety of structures which would require technically difficult and physiologically crippling operations for their removal. In addition, there may be spread via the blood stream, to the liver and the lungs, and across the peritoneal cavity (*transcoelomic*) to produce deposits in any part of the visceral or parietal peritoneum but particularly in the pouch of Douglas (between the rectum and uterus or bladder). It is this tendency to widespread dissemination that makes the condition so lethal and operation so ineffectual at producing cure.

Nevertheless, there is some hope for the future, in the concept pioneered in

Japan, of the 'early' gastric cancer. The term 'early' in this context means that the lesion is confined to the mucosa and submucosa, not *necessarily* (there is no evidence one way or the other) that it has only been present a short time. In Japan the combination of the impetus of a very high incidence of the disease with expertise in the manufacture of optical instruments led to an early development of the British invention of fibreoptics and the large-scale application of endoscopy to population-screening techniques for carcinoma of the stomach. This has led to the finding of many cases of early cancer, and gastrectomy has resulted in 5-year cure rates higher than 90 per cent in such patients. Presumably this means that widespread dissemination does not occur while the tumour is confined to the mucosa and submucosa. Recently, workers outside Japan have begun to produce similar excellent results.

Treatment

The only form of treatment that provides any hope of cure is surgery. The abdomen is opened and the presence of the carcinoma confirmed. The surgeon then has to decide the answer to two questions: (1) is the lesion resectable? and (2) is there any hope of cure? The tumour is not resectable if, for example, it is invading the pancreas; in such patients the abdomen is closed without any definitive procedure, although if gastric outlet obstruction has already developed or looks imminent it may be possible to perform a bypass (gastroenterostomy) between the stomach proximal to the tumour and the intestines beyond. If the tumour is resectable, it should be resected even if widespread metastases demonstrate that cure cannot be hoped for; the best palliation, with respect to pain, nausea and vomiting, is provided by removal of the main tumour mass.

Operations aiming at cure fall into two groups (Fig. 3.10). For lesions in the lower half of the stomach, an extensive partial (subtotal) gastrectomy is

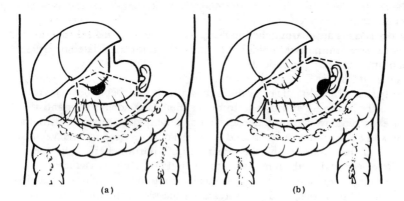

(a)   (b)

Fig. 3.10 Operations for removal of carcinoma of the stomach. (a) Radical partial gastrectomy for carcinoma of the antrum. The whole of the greater omentum and most of the lesser omentum are removed with the distal two-thirds of the stomach. (b) Radical total gastrectomy for carcinoma of the body or fundus. In addition to the whole stomach, the lower oesophagus and the two omenta, the spleen and tail of pancreas are removed as well.

performed with removal of the lesser and greater omenta and the related lymph nodes. For lesions higher in the stomach, any operation less than total gastrectomy is likely to fail because the line of excision of the stomach wall may not clear of the tumour: there is a marked tendency to submucosal spread of the growth, not visible to the naked eye. Total gastrectomy can be performed via the abdomen, but it is technically easier to achieve good clearance by a combined abdominothoracic approach, in which event the spleen and tail of pancreas are removed in a single block with the stomach and omenta.

Cytotoxic agents have been tried extensively in this disease, with disappointing results. However, 5-fluorouracil (5-FU) and mitomycin have been of some use in the palliation of symptoms from inoperable carcinoma. *Radiotherapy* is little used because of the sensitivity of neighbouring structures to x-rays.

Carcinoma of the pancreas

Pancreatic exocrine adenocarcinoma is now the second most common abdominal malignancy, and its incidence is increasing while that of gastric carcinoma declines. The cause of this phenomenon is unknown.

Aetiology
As in the case of gastric carcinoma, there is strong evidence that the main aetiological factors are environmental. The incidence of pancreatic carcinoma in Japanese who have immigrated into the United States is higher (approaching the native American figures) than in Japanese in Japan, and a strong association with cigarette-smoking has been reported from several centres. Weaker associations seem to exist with a high fat diet, a previous history of cholecystectomy, diabetes mellitus and working in the chemical manufacturing industry. Genetic factors may be important also: the incidence in Maoris is much higher than in other New Zealanders, and in black Americans than in white.

The sex ratio is approximately 2 males to every 1 female, and the incidence rises with age until, by 75 years, it is eight times that of the general population.

Clinical picture
The directly related symptoms, apart from jaundice, produced by an advanced carcinoma of the pancreas are pain and (much less commonly) steatorrhoea. The pain is upper abdominal, usually with radiation through to the back. Characteristically it is aggravated by lying down and relieved by bending forwards. A patient who squats because he finds that position provides some relief usually has pancreatic (or pericardial) disease. The pain may be due to the invasion of nerves in the posterior abdominal wall, because it is similar to that produced by the rapid enlargement of an aortic aneurysm; it may also be due to the damming back of exocrine secretion behind a neoplastic stricture of the main duct. Because of this latter possible mechanism, the pain may be aggravated by eating and this may lead to a misdiagnosis of 'dyspepsia, possibly due to a peptic ulcer'. If there is so little

pancreatic exocrine secretion reaching the duodenum that the digestion and therefore the absorption of fat is impaired, steatorrhoea results—the stools are frequent, loose, bulky, greasy in appearance, and float rather than sink in water. (For the investigation of pancreatic exocrine function, see p. 46.) Weight loss is an important feature, and due to the combination of pain and anorexia with malabsorption; occasionally, diabetes mellitus is a factor.

One clinical feature which, while rare, occurs sufficiently frequently in association with carcinoma of the pancreas to require noting is recurrent thrombophlebitis of the lower limb—*thrombophlebitis migrans*. Malignant disease anywhere predisposes to venous thrombosis, but the mechanism is unknown.

Diagnosis

Nowadays, provided that the possibility of carcinoma of the pancreas is entertained, the diagnosis is relatively easy to achieve.

Ultrasonography demonstrates a mass in the pancreas and distinguishes between a solid (tumour) and a liquid (cyst) swelling, and distortion of the

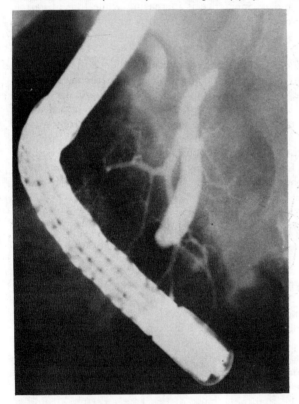

Fig. 3.11 Pancreatogram showing obstruction of the main duct. These appearances are typical of carcinoma of the pancreas. Contrast material injected into the pancreatic duct has outlined only the terminal few centimetres before being brought to an abrupt halt by a complete obstruction.

duct system by the mass is demonstrated by ERCP (Fig. 3.11). The focal nature of the lesion distinguishes carcinoma from the more widespread changes of chronic pancreatitis (p. 44). Other scanning techniques using radioactive isotopes are less accurate than ultrasonography, and though they have had their advocates they are being used less. A search for metastases includes a chest radiograph and possibly isotope scanning of the liver.

Treatment

Only surgical excision of the primary lesion with a wide margin, before metastasis has occurred beyond the field of operation, can cure this condition. Treatment by irradiation or chemotherapy offers no chance of cure and little effective palliation. The technical problems of surgery are formidable, and the known slender chances of achieving a cure must in each patient be balanced against the morbidity and mortality of the operation required.

Laparotomy is performed, and if no metastases are found the tumour is tested by a trial dissection for resectability. For lesions in the tail a distal pancreatectomy can be performed, for lesions in the head and neck of the

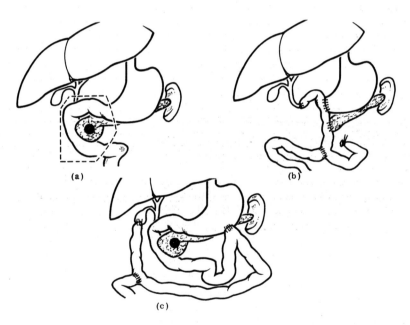

(a)

(b)

(c)

Fig. 3.12 (a and b). Whipple's operation of pancreatoduodenectomy for excision of carcinoma of the head of pancreas. (a) The extent of the excision is shown by dotted lines. (b) One method of reconstruction: a Roux loop of small intestine (see Fig. 2.5) is constructed and the cut proximal end of the common bile duct, of the gastric antrum and of the pancreas are inserted separately into the loop. (c) Bypass procedures for unresectable carcinoma of the pancreas. A Roux loop is attached to the distended gall bladder (or to the distended common bile duct if the cystic duct is of narrow calibre and the surgeon feels it might block). Since these tumours often obstruct the duodenum, a gastrojejunal anastomosis is often constructed as well.

organ a pancreatoduodenectomy (Whipple's operation), and for unresectable lesions the question of bypass procedures for palliation is considered (Fig. 3.12). Any suggestion of incipient obstruction to the duodenum leads to gastroenterostomy, of the biliary passages to an anastomosis between the gall bladder or the common bile duct on the one hand to the duodenum or jejunum on the other. The obstructed pancreatic duct can be drained by amputating the tail and inserting the stump into a loop of jejunum; however, the morbidity and mortality of this procedure are considerable, and satisfactory palliation of the pain is better achieved after operation by infiltration of the coeliac ganglion with local anaesthetic agents and destructive agents such as phenol.

Chronic pancreatitis

This uncommon disease derives disproportionate importance from the fact that its principal clinical feature is chronic (persistent) or intermittent upper abdominal pain. The diagnosis must therefore be carefully considered if investigation fails to uncover evidence of the more common causes of epigastric pain.

The exact *definition* of chronic pancreatitis is that it is an affection of the pancreas in which recurrent or persistent symptoms are associated with a demonstrable anatomical or functional abnormality of the pancreas even after any primary cause for the condition has been removed. The important distinction here is from recurrent acute pancreatitis (p. 108) in which the attacks of pain result from temporary obstruction of the terminal channel of the bile and pancreatic ducts by a passing gallstone or from the toxic effects of chronic overindulgence in alcohol but there is no demonstrable abnormality of the pancreas between attacks.

Aetiology
Chronic alcoholism is by far the most important factor in continental Europe and North America, and with the increase in consumption of alcohol in the United Kingdom in recent years the prevalence of the disease is increasing there also. In the tropics (South-east Asia and parts of Africa) the disease is much more common than anywhere else and is associated with *malnutrition* due to deficiency of protein and calories. *Hypercalcaemia* is a rare but clear-cut factor. A genetic predisposition certainly exists in that a *familial* variety of chronic pancreatitis has been described (some patients have mucoviscidosis, as well as chronic pancreatitis), and also an association with the genetically determined *alpha-1-antitrypsin* deficiency (p. 91). The vexed question is whether disease of the biliary tract (i.e. gallstones), acting via the passage of stones down the common duct and thus causing inflammation and stricture of the termination of the pancreatic duct, is a frequent cause. If it were, then there would be an association between acute or recurrent acute pancreatitis on the one hand and chronic pancreatitis on the other. Partly because the finer points of the pathology of chronic pancreatitis are not widely appreciated, there is still controversy about this; however, obstruction of the termination of the main

pancreatic duct produces very different pathological features from those of chronic pancreatitis.

Pathology
The primary disturbance appears to be the formation in the finer pancreatic ducts of plugs consisting of protein. The plugs result from precipitation of pancreatic enzymes, due to an increased concentration (i.e. rate of production) of enzymes or to the presence of some factor that reduces the solubility of the enzymes. Lactoferrin, which is present in the secretions of pancreas in patients with disease but not in normal pancreatic juice, may be such a factor. Hypercalcaemia promotes the secretion of protein-rich pancreatic juice.

The plugs become attached to the walls of the fine ducts and the latter become obstructed. The acinus in relation to an obstructed duct collapses, and becomes the seat of chronic inflammation with acute episodes, these changes gradually spreading through the neighbouring parenchyma to involve neighbouring islets of Langerhans. At a late stage, large protein plugs form in the main pancreatic duct, producing a series of strictures, often with calcification, at various points. This late involvement of the main duct is the distinction from the picture resulting from the traumatic passage of a common duct gallstone.

Dilatation of a large duct proximal to a major site of obstruction may lead to the formation of a cyst. If the latter bursts through the parenchyma, the resultant cavity—lined mostly with granulation tissue on the surface of surrounding organs such as stomach, omentum or colon—is called a pancreatic pseudocyst.

Clinical features
The predominant symptom is *pain*, usually upper abdominal and intermittent, but sometimes persistent and occasionally lower abdominal. Radiation to the back is common, and the squatting sign (p. 41) is rarely encountered but very characteristic of pancreatic pain. Patients can sometimes localize their pain accurately to the side, right or left, of pain that originates in localized disease. The cause of the pain is often unknown, although obstruction of a major pancreatic duct produces very severe and unrelenting pain. Rich (greasy) food and alcohol commonly produce a severe exacerbation, and the patient becomes afraid to eat and thus *loses weight*.

The symptoms have usually been present for many years before pancreatic insufficiency—endocrine or exocrine—develops. *Diabetes mellitus* is presumably due to interference with the production of insulin disproportionately more than with the production of glucagon, but it has been difficult to prove this thesis by measuring the output of these hormones in response, say, to a carbohydrate meal. *Pancreatic exocrine deficiency* does not develop until the ability of the pancreas to secrete its digestive enzymes has been reduced to about 10 per cent of normal.

The principal feature of pancreatic insufficiency is *steatorrhoea*, the passage of large, pale and often frothy stools, these features being due mainly to the high content of undigested fat in the stools. On an average hospital ward diet, the fat content of the patient's faeces measured over a 3-day period should normally not exceed 5 g per day. Any excess can be used as a working definition of steatorrhoea. The cause is the deficiency of pancreatic lipase, and this is the *only* cause that can produce very severe degrees of steatorrhoea, that is of the order of 50 g fat per day.

The interference with the absorption of fat reduces the absorption of the fat-soluble vitamins A, D and K, but very rarely to an extent that gives rise to a clinical disturbance. Similarly, protein malabsorption can often be demonstrated by special tests, and gives rise to wasting of muscle but only very rarely to hypoalbuminaemia and oedema.

Cysts and pseudocysts may cause pain by pressure on neighbouring structures, and may grow to great size. They may also produce venous obstruction in the portal system and thus haematemesis from oesophageal varices (p. 128).

Diagnosis

At a late stage, a plain x-ray of the upper abdomen frequently reveals calcification. This is usually confined to the ducts, where the protein plugs calcify, but it may extend into the parenchyma.

Deficiency of pancreatic exocrine secretion can be investigated by any of several standard tests in which the duodenal contents are aspirated (the stomach is aspirated at the same time to minimize contamination with gastric juice) and analysed for bicarbonate and/or pancreatic enzymes after stimulation of the pancreas by a standard meal or an injection of secretin and

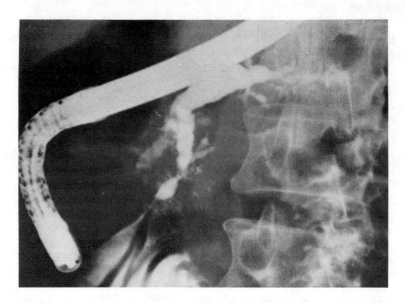

Fig. 3.13 Pancreatogram obtained by ERCP in a patient with chronic pancreatitis. Note the irregularities of the wall of the duct, with strictured zones interspersed with dilated areas.

pancreozymin. The principle underlying the use of bicarbonate outputs and concentrations is that bile and succus entericus cannot secrete bicarbonate in greater concentration than about 25 mmol/l (25 mEq/l) but that the stimulated pancreas can normally achieve a concentration of 140–150 mmol/l (Sanford: *Digestive System Physiology*, Chapter 4). Thus the bicarbonate in duodenal contents reflects the secretory ability of the pancreas much more than the response of the other sources.

The technique of ERCP (p. 36) allows the pancreatic duct to be cannulated, and so it has become possible for pure pancreatic juice to be collected. Though one might expect this technique to yield more accurate data for identifying chronic pancreatitis, recent work suggests that the diseased gland secretes bicarbonate at a fairly normal concentration but the volume of juice secreted is abnormally low. Since the accurate measurement of the volume of the pure juice is much more difficult than the measurement of bicarbonate concentration, studies with pure juice have proved disappointing. However, much more important is the ability to use the cannulation of the pancreatic duct for injecting radio-opaque contrast material, so outlining the duct system and obtaining an accurate picture of strictures, dilatations (including cysts and pseudocysts), and space-occupying lesions within the parenchyma (Fig. 3.13).

Treatment
Pain is the over-riding consideration. Alcohol is forbidden for ever, and complete abstinence greatly reduces the severity of attacks although it does not guarantee complete relief. Analgesics also help: acetylsalicyclic acid should be avoided because it can increase any tendency to haematemesis, but paracetamol and dextropropoxyphene are useful. A low fat diet may help. In patients with severe and debilitating pain, blocking the autonomic afferents from the pancreas at the coeliac axis (p. 44) is well worth while; a good result may last several months and can be repeated. For the hard core of remaining sufferers, various surgical procedures are available although these tend to be complicated and dangerous. Cysts and pseudocysts are drained internally, usually into the stomach; the main pancreatic duct can be drained proximal to the major site of obstruction by laying open the duct through an incision on the anterior aspect of the pancreas and anastomosing the duct to a loop of jejunum. Finally, various forms of pancreatectomy are practised, from a local resection of a limited lesion ranging through resection of the head of pancreas (Whipple's operation) and subtotal pancreatectomy (leaving a thin rim of pancreas on the convexity of the duodenum), to total pancreatectomy in which, as in Whipple's procedure, the pyloric antrum and duodenal loop must be removed (see Fig. 3.12).

Pancreatic insufficiency arises either because of the disease or because of pancreatectomy for pain. *Diabetes mellitus* is usually mild if it is the disease alone that is responsible; after total or subtotal pancreatectomy, insulin will be necessary. Exocrine insufficiency is treated by a low fat (30 g per day) diet with extra carbohydrate given as readily assimilable small molecules, not as starch, and with preparations of pancreatic enzymes. Because these enzymes are acid-labile, it seems logical to reduce gastric acid secretion in an effort to ensure that a greater proportion of the enzyme preparation reaches the duodenum, and encouraging results have recently been reported using cimetidine (p. 57).

Further reading

Hand, B. H. (1976). Presentation and management of stones in the common bile duct. In *Current Surgical Practice,* vol. 1, pp. 114–132. Ed. by G. J. Hadfield and M. Hobsley. Edward Arnold, London.

Cotton, P. B. and Williams, C. B. (1980). *Practical Gastrointestinal Endoscopy.* Blackwell Scientific, Oxford.

Go, V. L. W. and DiMagno, E. P. (1977). Pancreatic exocrine adenocarcinoma. *British Journal of Hospital Medicine* **18**, 567–576.

Hatfield, A. R. W. (1977). The investigation of pancreatic exocrine disorders. *British Journal of Hospital Medicine* **18**, 528–545.

Johnston, D. (1976). Modern Surgical Attitudes to Peptic Ulceration. In *Current Surgical Practice,* vol. 1, pp. 73–113. Ed. by G. J. Hadfield and M. Hobsley. Edward Arnold, London.

Kaneko, E., Nakamura, T., Umeda, N., Fujino, M. and Niwa, H. (1977). Outcome of gastric carcinoma detected by gastric mass survey in Japan. *Gut* **18**, 626–630.

Longmire, W. P. (1980). Gastric carcinoma: is radical gastrectomy worth while? *Annals of the Royal College of Surgeons of England* **62**, 25–30.

Mallinson, C. (1977). Chronic pancreatitis. *British Journal of Hospital Medicine* **18**, 553–566.

Polk, H. C. Jr and Zeppa, R. (1971). Hiatal hernia and esophagitis: a survey of indications for operation and technique and results of fundoplication. *Annals of Surgery* **173**, 775–781.

Price, W. H. (1963). Gallbladder dyspepsia. *British Medical Journal* **2**, 138–141.

Rogers, I. M., Moule, B. Sokhi, G. S., Joffe, S. N. and Blumgart, L. H. (1976). Endoscopy and routine and double-contrast barium meal in diagnosis of gastric and duodenal disorders. *Lancet* **1**, 901–902.

Schiller, K. F. R. (ed.) (1978). *Endoscopy. Clinics in Gastroenterology* **7**, no. 3.

Trapnell, J. E. (1976). Pancreatitis: acute and chronic. In *Current Surgical Practice,* vol. 1, pp. 132–148. Ed. by G. J. Hadfield and M. Hobsley. Edward Arnold, London.

4

Peptic ulcer:
aetiology and management

The incidence of chronic peptic ulceration has undergone interesting changes. During the nineteenth century it was probably rare, although, without modern methods of investigation, it is difficult to be sure. During the first two decades of the present century, gastric ulcer was the common lesion and presented most commonly in young women. Since the 1930s duodenal ulcer has become, relative to gastric ulcer and also absolutely, much more common and the typical patient with a chronic duodenal ulcer is now a man aged 40–50 years while benign gastric ulceration predominantly occurs in men and women older than 60 years.

Phenomena such as these indicate that the aetiology of peptic ulcer disease must be complex, changing, and probably different between duodenal and gastric ulcer. Moreover, duodenal ulcer is very common. The prevalence of peptic ulcer in the population of the United Kingdom is about 6 per cent: at any one moment, 3 million out of about 50 million people have the disease. Many of them have symptoms, so this is a staggering clinical load.

Aetiology

Whatever other factors may be important in producing peptic ulcers, the presence of acid–pepsin secreted by the stomach is crucial. The site of peptic ulcers, at or near the junction between acid- and alkaline-secreting mucosa, was commented upon on Chapter 3. The core of the relationship between gastric acid secretion and peptic ulceration can be summarized in the phrase: 'No acid—no ulcer'. No authentic case of peptic ulcer has been described in an individual who was incapable of secreting hydrochloric acid from his gastric mucosa (p. 53).

Three other lines of evidence link the peptic ulcer diathesis with gastric secretion. First, patients whose stomachs are driven all the time, even under apparently basal conditions, to secrete large quantities of gastric juice, approaching the amounts that they would secrete under maximal stimulation, suffer from a particularly intractable form of peptic ulceration called the Zollinger–Ellison syndrome (p. 61). Secondly, patients with duodenal ulcer (not gastric ulcer) tend *as a group* to have greater basal and maximal secretion than do control groups. Thirdly, any measures that reduce the capacity of the parietal cells to secrete acid, whether they be medical (p. 57) or surgical (p. 58), produce healing of the ulcer.

Rates of secretion of hydrochloric acid and of pepsin usually run closely parallel, and pepsin is much more complicated to measure than hydrochloric acid. For these reasons, less attention has been paid to pepsin than to acid, and this chapter concentrates mainly on measurements of acid (although see p. 56).

Tests of gastric acid secretion

The concept that one subject makes more gastric acid than another is deceptively simple. Quantitative assessment requires consideration of many factors.

Secretogogue

Isolated parietal cells in tissue culture secrete hydrochloric acid in response to acetylcholine, gastrin (p. 61) and histamine. In a human with an intact stomach, gastrin and histamine seem in quantitative terms to be equivalent stimuli in that when a sufficiently high dose of each of these agents is given, the gastric secretory response reaches an identical maximal rate. The present evidence suggests that the response to acetylcholine, while proportionate to the maximal response, only reaches 80–90 per cent of the maximum.

In normal circumstances (Sanford: *Digestive System Physiology*, Chapter 3) acetylcholine is released near parietal cells as a result of stimulation of the vagus nerve ('appetite juice' at the sight and smell of food—later, the response of afferents from the gastric mucosa when the food reaches there), while the hormone *gastrin* is released from the gastrin-secreting cells (G cells) of the antrum in response to the *chemical* presence within the stomach of non-fatty foods, particularly proteins. The appetite-juice element of the vagal pathway can be stimulated by sham-feeding (the subject smells, tastes and chews food but then spits it out without swallowing), and the whole vagal pathway by producing hypoglycaemia (usually with insulin), which stimulates the vagal centres in the medulla. The chemical pathway can be stimulated by a protein-rich meal, by gastrin or synthetic analogues of gastrin, and by histamine.

One way of reducing the ability of the stomach to secrete acid is by the operation of *abdominal vagotomy*, dividing the abdominal vagi proximal to the stomach; insulin hypoglycaemia has therefore been the common method of testing gastric secretion *after* this operation. Testing *before* any operation has usually been performed with pentagastrin, a synthetic analogue of gastrin, or with histamine, since these agents can be used to stimulate maximal secretion and the output of acid produced has been shown to be related to the number of parietal cells contained in that individual's stomach. Whichever mechanism is being tested, the end-response for measurement is the amount and/or acidity of the gastric juice secreted, and it is therefore convenient that all these secretogogues are given parenterally so that the stomach of the (fasting) individual contains only the juice it has secreted: this can be collected by aspiration via a nasogastric tube.

The objection can be raised that the gastric response to such artificial stimuli may differ from its response to normal food. An ingenious technique has recently been devised to measure the response to a normal meal. The subject eats the meal with a nasogastric tube in position, and decinormal sodium hydroxide is instilled simultaneously via one channel of the tube. Small samples of the stomach contents are aspirated at intervals and their pH determined. The rate of instillation of the alkali is varied so as to maintain the reaction of the stomach contents as constant as possible; under these circumstances, the rate of addition of alkali must be the same as the rate of secretion of acid by the stomach. Sufficient experience has not yet been gained with this technique to establish normal standards.

If one assumes that the parietal cell response to endogenous gastrin is normal, information about the chemical pathway can be obtained from the rise in plasma gastrin concentration after a standard meal. Commercial meat extracts have been used, but the G cell response seems to be greater with ordinary food and attempts have been made to establish a 'standard English breakfast'. The difficulty with this approach is that the measurement of gastrin by the radioimmunoassay technique is available only at special centres and is subject to considerable error.

Route and dose

Hypoglycaemia is usually produced with soluble insulin, 0.2 units/kg, by intravenous bolus dose (Table 4.1), although an intravenous infusion technique has also been advocated.

Table 4.1 Secretogogues used in gastric secretion studies

Active agent	Preparation	Bolus dose	IV infusion dose
Histamine	Acid phosphate Dihydrochloride	40 μg/kg 50 μg/kg	$40\ \mu g \cdot kg^{-1} \cdot h^{-1}$
Pentagastrin		6 μg/kg	$6\ \mu g \cdot kg^{-1} \cdot h^{-1}$
Insulin	Soluble	2 units/kg (IV)	

The *chemical pathway* is tested with pentagastrin or histamine given by a one-shot or continuous intravenous infusion technique, in the dosages described in Table 4.1. Pentagastrin can be given in this dosage with relatively few side-effects, but the unpleasant flushing, headache, nasal congestion and bronchospasm produced by histamine demand prior medication with an H1-blocker (Sanford: *Digestive System Physiology*, Chapter 3) such as mepyramine maleate (Anthisan). The recommended doses of these secretogogues have been shown to elicit the maximal possible rate of secretion.

Collection and estimation

Gastric secretion is aspirated continuously via the nasogastric tube, though the aspirate may be divided into separate 10- or 15-minute collections. The first half hour of a collection to determine *basal* secretion is rejected, because it takes this length of time for the secretion to settle down to the basal state after the stimulus of swallowing the tube. The first half hour following the injection of insulin in a test of the vagal mechanism is also rejected, because the direct action of insulin itself on gastric secretion is one of slight depression until the blood sugar has fallen sufficiently to stimulate the vagal centres. After any such preliminary period has been completed, the collection period is at least 1 hour in most tests, and 1½ hours in the insulin test.

The method of estimation usually used is to titrate an aliquot of each sample of gastric juice to an end-point of pH 7, thus determining the titratable acidity in mmol (mEq) per litre. Sodium measurements are useful in determining duodenogastric reflux (see below).

Expression of results

The standard method is to multiply the hydrogen ion concentration in each sample by the volume of the sample to get hydrogen ion output, and this output is then expressed in mmol per hour. Secretion during a basal hour is called *basal acid output* (BAO). The total acid output during the hour following histamine or pentagastrin in maximal dosage is called the *maximal acid output* (MAO). In such one-shot studies, the rate of secretion is rising in the early stages and falling in the late, with the true maximal rate being achieved in the middle. A more accurate representation of maximal secretory activity is therefore achieved by collecting in 10- or 15-minute samples, noting the acid output in the total of two or three samples in a consecutive 30 minutes in which the acid output was maximal, and multiplying by two to give the hourly rate of *peak acid output* (PAO). Best of all, the rate at which secretion stabilizes during a continuous intravenous infusion of the secretogogue, the *plateau maximal acid output* (MAOpl), is usually about 10 per cent higher than PAO. In insulin tests, it would appear that the best methods of expressing the results are as peak or average acid output per hour, during the period ½–2 hours after the injection.

Collection errors

The chief sources of error are pyloric losses, duodenogastric reflux and swallowed saliva. There is at present no satisfactory method for preventing, or correcting for, saliva. Pyloric losses can be quantified with the aid of a non-absorbable marker (Fig. 4.1): the dilution of the marker permits calculation of the volume into which it has been diluted. Duodenogastric reflux contains sodium ions in a concentration of 150 mmol/l (150 mEq/l), compared with much smaller concentrations (10–40 mmol/l) in gastric juice. Measurement of the sodium concentration of the aspirate allows the reflux to be quantified. These correction techniques are not standard, but seem to increase accuracy.

Secretion norms

Maximal secretion is related to stature. In general, adults can secrete more rapidly than children, while the taller races of Western Europe and North America secrete more rapidly than the shorter natives of South-east Asia. Secretion, in the adult, diminishes with age, although the effect is small. Sex has no effect, after allowing for the link between sex and stature. An important recent finding is that smoking cigarettes seems to increase maximal gastric secretion: there was a positive correlation between maximal secretion and the total number of cigarettes smoked in a control group of 84 subjects in London. The relation of this finding to the aetiology of duodenal ulcer is considered later.

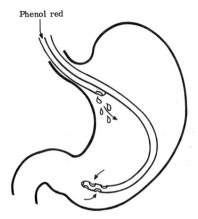

Phenol red

Fig. 4.1 Principle of using a non-absorbable marker to quantify the volume of gastric juice secreted by dye-dilution. The marker (e.g. phenol red) is infused into the upper part of the stomach through the shorter lumen of the double-lumen nasogastric tube. After mixing in the gastric juice, the marker is aspirated through the longer lumen. The degree of dilution of the marker in the aspirate measures the volume of secretion into which the marker has been diluted, irrespective of whether or not any secretion has been lost via the pylorus.

Acid secretion and peptic ulcer: quantitative aspects

Achlorhydria

The most clear-cut practical use of gastric secretion studies is to demonstrate achlorhydria—the inability of an individual to secrete hydrochloric acid. Achlorhydria can only be diagnosed if a maximal form of stimulus has been used, i.e. histamine or pentagastrin. Achlorhydria is incompatible with a diagnosis of peptic ulcer, and so a gastric ulcer in a patient shown to be achlorhydric must be neoplastic. This can be useful evidence if endoscopic biopsy of a gastric ulcer has failed to confirm a clinical suspicion of carcinoma.

In most patients with achlorhydria, the defect has developed as a result of atrophic gastritis affecting the parietal cell area, and there is an associated inability to secrete intrinsic factor (Sanford: *Digestive System Physiology*, Chapter 3). In consequence, these patients are unable to absorb vitamin B_{12} (cyanocobalamin) and in time develop pernicious anaemia unless treated with parenteral injections of B_{12}. However, achlorhydria may occasionally be found in young people as a genetically determined disorder, without atrophic gastritis, and such subjects, although their production of intrinsic factor is much impaired, always secrete enough to prevent the onset of pernicious anaemia.

Duodenal ulcer

Figure 4.2 shows some recently published data. After standardization for height, patients with duodenal ulcer had a significantly greater mean V_G (gastric secretory volume corrected for pyloric losses and duodenogastric reflux) than the control group. Further standardization for cigarette-smoking

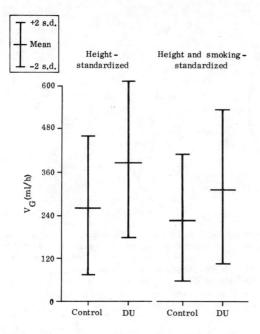

Fig. 4.2 Maximal secretion in a control group and a group of patients with duodenal ulcer. The acid data are corrected for pyloric losses and duodenogastric reflux (called V_G here) and standardized for height. They are shown with and without standardization of cigarette-smoking. *See text* for full discussion.

reduced this difference by about two-thirds, but the residual difference was still significant. The other important point is that, in terms of height-standardized secretion, only 25 per cent of the duodenal ulcer patients had a maximal secretion greater than the 95 per cent tolerance limits of the control group. Therefore only in this minority could hypersecretion be a *sole* aetiological factor for duodenal ulcer. Moreover, it would appear that cigarette-smoking could account for two-thirds of this hypersecretion (95 per cent of the duodenal ulcer group were habitual smokers, compared with only 50 per cent of the control group), but that the remaining one-third of the hypersecretion must be due to some other factor. Finally, in the three-quarters of the duodenal ulcer patients whose maximal secretion rates were within the boundaries of the control group, any tendency towards hypersecretion could not be the *sole* cause of the disease but might summate with other aetiological factors.

Gastric ulcer
It seems quite clear that there is no tendency to hypersecretion in patients with gastric ulcer. Indeed, there is some tendency to hyposecretion, though not enought to be useful in diagnosis (apart from histamine-fast achlorhydria).

Zollinger–Ellison syndrome

This syndrome (p. 61) is due to an excess of circulating gastrin, derived usually from a tumour of G cells in the pancreas. In consequence, even under apparently basal conditions the stomachs of sufferers secrete actively. Studies have not yet been reported taking collection errors into account, but height is not important as each subject acts as his own control, his 'basal' secretion being compared with his maximal. Table 4.2 shows the generally accepted criteria for making the diagnosis. Note that *maximal* hypersecretion is not part of the criteria.

Table 4.2 Generally accepted gastric secretory criteria for diagnosis of Zollinger-Ellison syndrome

Index of secretion	Diagnostic range
Basal acid output	> 15 mmol in 1 h (intact stomach) > 5 mmol/h (postoperative)
12-hour nocturnal secretion	> 1000 ml or > 100 ml/h
Ratio $\dfrac{\text{basal acid output}}{\text{maximal acid output}}$	> 0.6
Ratio $\dfrac{\text{basal titratable acidity}}{\text{maximal titratable acidity}}$	> 0.6

Acid and ulcer: a summary

Certain general conclusions can be drawn. First, *some* acid–pepsin must be being secreted if peptic ulceration is to occur. Secondly, if the total amount of acid–pepsin secreted increases sufficiently, either because the number of parietal cells increases (maximal secretion above the normal range) or because the parietal cells are secreting maximally all the time (Zollinger–Ellison), duodenal ulceration occurs. Thirdly, the increased parietal cell mass is largely, but not completely, associated quantitatively with cigarette-smoking. Fourthly, in the majority of patients with peptic ulcer, gastric secretion is in the normal range and so some other aetiological factor or factors must be present (although their influence may be enhanced by the tendency to an increase in parietal cell mass related to smoking).

Other factors

The changes in the epidemiology of duodenal ulcer commented on at the beginning of this chapter fit quite well the statistics for cigarette-smoking. The vast increase in cigarette-smoking after the 1914–18 war corresponded with an increased prevalence of duodenal ulcers from the 1930s. However, patients with gastric ulcer show no hypersecretion and neither do most patients with duodenal ulcer.

Several other factors have been shown to be statistically associated with peptic ulcer disease. Patients with duodenal ulcer are said to be of blood group O and of positive blood group secretor status more often than would be expected by chance; whereas patients with gastric ulcer tend to have blood group A. The HLA antigens B5 and B12 have been reported to be associated with peptic ulcer. The female sex seems to exert a protective effect since patients with duodenal ulcer are so much more frequently male than female. There also appear to be differences in the types and quantity of pepsinogen and pepsin secreted by ulcer subjects. Finally, with regard to gastric ulcer, suggested aetiological factors include smoking (which would presumably act in some way other than through hypersecretion of acid–pepsin, since there is none), alcohol, chronic gastritis, reflux of duodenal contents (particularly bile) into the stomach associated presumably with incompetence of the pylorus, and certain drugs (such as acetylsalicylic acid, corticosteroids, phenylbutazone) which apparently destroy the gastric mucosal barrier and permit the gastric secretions to diffuse back into the mucosa and attack it.

Management

Strategy

Peptic ulceration is a chronic disease with acute exacerbations and acute complications. Its overall natural history is unknown, although there is some evidence for duodenal ulcer that the disease may become quiescent—'burn itself out'—after 15–20 years. In between the periods of exacerbation, the patient may be symptomless—sometimes for long periods. Management therefore involves, on the one hand, the control of symptoms during exacerbations, and on the other, measures designed to influence the natural history and cut it short. Important further considerations are that the complications—bleeding, perforation and stenosis (Chapter 7)—are life-threatening, and that a gastric ulcer might be an as yet unrecognized carcinoma.

Treatment is discussed under three headings, symptomatic, histamine H2-receptor blockade, and curative.

Symptomatic

The cause of pain is by no means clear-cut (Chapter 3). However, the typical relationship of the pain to meals and its response to antacids have led to the assumption that the pain is due to hydrochloric acid (and pepsin) acting on the surface of the raw ulcer. The mainstay of symptomatic treatment is therefore antacids, although many physicians also prescribe anticholinergics such as atropine and propantheline since these can be shown temporarily to reduce secretion by their blocking effect on the vagal terminals. The relief produced by antacids can be dramatically rapid, and the symptoms, once relieved, usually do not return for several hours.

As long as they keep the patient's life tolerable, symptomatic measures can be continued. Even so, the absence of symptoms does not necessarily mean that the ulcer has healed. The longer a patient has an ulcer, the greater becomes the chance of complications such as bleeding, perforation or stenosis. Thus as time passes, and certainly if the symptoms cannot be controlled, the necessity for curative measures increases. How long one should persist with symptomatic measures depends on many factors: the severity of symptoms, the frequency of attacks, the degree of interference with work and leisure, but perhaps most clearly the site of the ulcer, whether duodenal or gastric. For practical purposes, a duodenal ulcer is never malignant, whereas carcinoma of the stomach is common, is often difficult to distinguish from a benign ulcer and in some cases may develop in the edge of a benign ulcer. A gastric ulcer should undergo endoscopic biopsy, and, if it does not heal after a full course of medical treatment (next paragraph) or if it recurs after having healed, laparotomy should be undertaken.

Apart from measures which definitely reduce the ability of the stomach to secrete acid–pepsin, the only factors that have been shown to influence the rate of healing of a peptic ulcer are bed-rest and the cessation of smoking. Both gastric and duodenal ulcers respond. Gastric ulcers definitely, duodenal ulcers possibly, also heal quicker in ambulant patients if the drug carbenoxolone is given, but this agent does not further enhance the rate of healing in patients at rest in bed. The mechanisms whereby bed-rest and carbenoxolone work are unknown, but the last-named has important side-effects associated with its corticosteroid-like property of retaining water: hypertension may ensue. Presumably, stopping smoking works by a reduction of its effect enhancing gastric secretion, but this mechanism has not been substantiated. Clinicians also usually advise the patient to reduce his consumption of alcohol, although this is empirical.

Histamine H2-receptor blockers

A class of drugs has recently been discovered that blocks the action of histamine on the parietal cell. The most effective of these in general use is cimetidine. In a regimen of 200 mg three times a day plus 400 mg at bedtime, about 90 per cent of patients with peptic ulcer get rapid relief of symptoms, and gastric secretion in response to 'maximal' doses of histamine and pentagastrin is reduced in about 85 per cent of cases to about 40 per cent of the pretreatment value.

There is no doubt that in most cases this is a highly effective regimen for producing rapid healing of a peptic ulcer. The natural history of patients when they stop taking the drug is becoming clear. Some 75 per cent of patients relapse, and so far attempts to keep the ulcer healed on a modified regimen of smaller dosage for many months have not yielded very encouraging results in that, as soon as acid secretion is allowed to return to pretreatment levels, about 75 per cent develop a recurrence of their duodenal ulcer.

The drug has a special place for the treatment of those patients with the Zollinger–Ellison syndrome (p. 61).

Surgical operations

Duodenal and gastric ulcers must be considered separately, because of the ever-present possibility of malignancy in a gastric ulcer.

For duodenal ulcers, the popular operations at present are partial gastrectomy, some form of vagotomy, or a combination of both types. All these operations have in common the fact that they reduce the capacity of the stomach or gastric remnant to secrete acid. Interruption of the vagal pathways reduces insulin-stimulated secretion practically to basal levels, and even histamine-stimulated secretion is reduced to about 40 per cent of normal. In the operation of partial gastrectomy, the pylorus and pyloric antrum are removed to eliminate the major source of gastrin (although there are some G cells in the duodenum and even further down the small intestine), but the

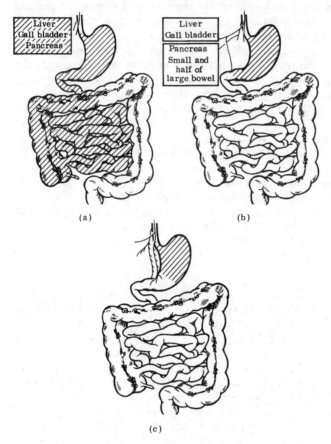

(a)   (b)

(c)

Fig. 4.3 Types of vagotomy. Vagally denervated areas are shaded.   (a) *Truncal.* Division of the two main trunks of the vagus at the lower end of the oesophagus vagally denervates the liver, gall bladder and pancreas as well as the stomach, small bowel, and large bowel as far as the mid-transverse colon (shaded).   (b) *Selective.* The left or anterior vagus is divided after it has given off hepatic branches to the liver and gall bladder (and one to the pylorus); the right or posterior vagus is divided after it has given off a coeliac branch to the pancreas and bowel. The whole stomach (but perhaps not the pylorus itself) is vagally denervated.   (c) *Proximal gastric* (*highly selective*) preserves the main trunks and all their branches except the small ones supplying the parietal cell area of the stomach.

proximal limit of resection is much higher than the junction of body and antrum, the distal two-thirds or so of the stomach being removed. This procedure thus reduces the parietal cell mass, and it has been shown that the reduction in maximal secretion produced by the operation is related to the number of parietal cells in the resected portion of stomach.

Vagotomy is probably technically safer than partial gastrectomy, and intrinsically more attractive as a less mutilating operation. However, the vagus nerves are motor to the muscle of the stomach wall as well as secretomotor to the parietal cells and so some disturbance of the stomach emptying mechanism is to be anticipated after vagotomy. When the vagal nerve trunks are divided in the region of the lower end of the oesophagus (truncal vagotomy, Fig. 4.3a), some form of mechanical rearrangement to increase the rate of gastric emptying is therefore carried out (the so-called drainage procedure). This may take the form of destruction of the valvular mechanism of the pylorus (pyloroplasty) or of bypassing the pylorus (antroduodenostomy or gastroenterostomy).

Truncal vagotomy denervates not only the whole of the stomach, but also the liver, gall bladder, pancreas and intestines up to the region of the mid-transverse colon. While there are no known adverse *clinical* effects of this widespread denervation, it has been shown that the pancreatic ability to secrete glucagon in response to insulin hypoglycaemia, or bicarbonate in response to acidification of the duodenum, is impaired after vagotomy, and doubtless there are other penalties that have not yet been defined. The operation of selective vagotomy (Fig. 4.3b) was therefore introduced: the innervation of the pylorus itself is maintained by the pyloric branch given off from the hepatic branch, and reaching the pylorus via the lesser omentum near its free border, but the pyloric antrum loses its vagal supply. Therefore, the most recently introduced type of vagotomy (Fig. 4.3c) maintains the antral supply in the hope that there will then be less interference with gastric emptying (p. 67). This type has several names, of which the most popular are proximal gastric vagotomy, highly selective vagotomy or parietal cell vagotomy. There is no necessity for a drainage procedure after this operation, provided that fibrosis has not produced stenosis of the gastric outlet.

Gastroenterostomy
Historically the first operation introduced for the treatment of duodenal ulcer, gastroenterostomy is the only operation in which no attempt is made to reduce gastric secretion. The original rationale was to divert acid gastric contents away from the duodenum, but at least as important a factor is probably the reflux of large quantities of alkaline duodenal contents through the artificial stoma back into the stomach so that any gastric contents reaching the duodenum are far less acid.

Although this operation had considerable early success, it has now been virtually abandoned. The incidence of recurrent ulceration reaches unacceptable levels (more than 50 per cent) as the years pass after the operation, because the jejunal mucosa now exposed to the acid from the stomach is itself prone to peptic ulceration.

Adequacy of vagotomy

While gastric hypersecretion is certainly not essential for the production of a duodenal ulcer, the best evidence that gastric juice has something to do with the aetiology is that there is a close relationship after vagotomy between the level to which the gastric secretory ability has been reduced and the incidence of recurrent ulceration.

The classic approach to measuring the 'adequacy' of vagotomy is via the insulin test. Hollander suggested that a rise in hydrogen ion concentration in hypoglycaemia-stimulated gastric juice, compared with that in basal secretion just before the insulin was given, of 20 mmol/l or more, indicated an inadequate vagotomy—i.e. the patient would be likely to develop a recurrence of peptic ulceration. If the basal secretion was anacid, he suggested that the criterion sould be modified to a threshold value of only 10 mmol/l in the stimulated juice.

Although Hollander's criteria remain the most widely used, there has been dissatisfaction with their performance. Many modifications have been suggested but nearly all rely, as Hollander's did, on a comparison of insulin-stimulated secretion with basal secretion in the same patient. This ignores the physiological fact that basal secretion as usually measured (i.e. without correction for pyloric losses, etc.) is very variable, and that hydrogen ion concentration is particularly susceptible to the effects of duodenogastric reflux since the hydrogen ions are both diluted and neutralized by the alkaline regurgitation. The performance of the Hollander criteria can be improved by substituting for basal secretion as the index of comparison, insulin-stimulated secretion in patients with duodenal ulcer who have not undergone vagotomy, and then adding a number of refinements such as correction for collection errors and standardization for stature.

However, this approach to the problem has a flavour of shutting the stable door after the horse has bolted, since the operation has been completed long before it has been found to inadequate! The surgeon needs to know during the operation if his denervation is complete. Peroperative techniques to answer this question have been described. In one, gastric secretion is stimulated with an intravenous infusion of pentagastrin, and the surface of the stomach is explored with a pH probe introduced by the operator through a small incision in the stomach wall: before vagotomy the pH recorded from the parietal cell area is below 2, but after complete vagotomy no area has a pH below 6. In another technique, use is made of the fact that the vagus is not only secretomotor to the glands, but also motor to the muscle wall of the stomach. When the intragastric luminal pressure does not rise on stimulation of the vagus near the lower end of the oesophagus, vagotomy is complete. The use of such techniques would almost certainly reduce the incidence of recurrent ulceration after vagotomy, but they are difficult to apply and are used routinely in only a few centres.

Gastrin

The confirmation, many years after its existence was first postulated, that a hormone, gastrin, is involved in the chemical mechanism of gastric secretion led to hopes that alterations in gastrin metabolism or secretion rate might explain the pathogenesis of diseases that were apparently linked with alterations in gastric secretion. Except for one clinical condition, the Zollinger–Ellison syndrome, this expectation has not been realized. The interplay between gastrin and the other topics in this chapter is here briefly reviewed.

Duodenal ulcer

Acid hypersecretion by itself can be an aetiological factor in only about one-quarter of patients with duodenal ulceration. Certainly fasting gastrin concentrations in the plasma are normal or indeed low in patients with duodenal ulcers compared with normal subjects. This tendency to an inverse relationship may be explained by the relationship of plasma gastrin concentration to achlorhydria.

Achlorhydria

In patients with achlorhydria, the fasting plasma gastrin concentration is very high, of the order of 1000 pg/ml compared with the 0–50 pg/ml of normals. It appears that alkaline conditions in the stomach stimulate the G cells to produce gastrin, presumably in an effort to restore the medium to a more normal (acid) pH. Under the conditions of hyperacidity that occur *on average* in patients with duodenal ulcer, the reverse presumably occurs—the G cells are depressed.

The hypothesis of a reciprocal relationship between gastric acid secretion and G cell activity is supported by the finding that fasting plasma gastrin concentrations are high in individuals with hyposecretion of acid—patients with gastric ulcer, or who have undergone vagotomy or partial gastrectomy.

Zollinger–Ellison syndrome

The cardinal feature of this syndrome is an intractable ulcer diathesis, although some patients also complain of watery diarrhoea. In most patients, suspicion is aroused only when peptic ulceration recurs despite an apparently adequate, or even after a second, operation. However, there are some features suggestive of the diagnosis at the outset: multiple ulcers, ulcers situated distal to the usual site, (i.e. well beyond the first 2 cm of the duodenum) and hypertrophy of the gastric rugae as demonstrated in the barium meal.

The basal hypersecretion of acid typical of this syndrome has already been described (p. 55). It is due to an excessive secretion of gastrin from G cells that are autonomous; i.e. not subject to the normal inhibition produced by excess acid secretion. The diagnosis is confirmed by finding very high fasting plasma gastrin values—over 1000 pg/ml.

The gastrin, in nearly all cases, is secreted by one or more tumours of G cells in the pancreas. It is unwise to rely on excision of a palpable or visible pancreatic tumour as a cure for the condition, because there are so often more tumours present which cannot be detected. The standard approach has been to accept the tumours, and to remove the whole of their target organ—the stomach. This cures the ulcer diathesis, but the tumours are usually malignant and so the patient ultimately succumbs to widespread metastases. The advent of cimetidine has led to the possibility of controlling the hypersecretion and allowing the ulcers to heal, either as a long-term treatment or as a preparation for intensive investigation designed to demonstrate the site of the gastrinomas so that a direct surgical attack might become possible.

Gastrin in large concentrations increases bowel motility, and the diarrhoea experienced by some patients used to be ascribed to this factor. It has recently been shown, however, that the diarrhoea is more usually due to excess secretion by the tumour of a second hormone, vasoactive intestinal peptide (VIP), whose principal action is to produce diarrhoea. There are some patients who complain of the diarrhoea without peptic ulceration because their tumour produces VIP but no gastrin.

Further reading

Alexander-Williams, J. and Cox, A. G. (1969). *After Vagotomy.* Butterworths, London.

Baron, J. H. (1978). *Clinical Tests of Gastric Secretion: history, methodology and interpretation.* Macmillan, London.

Hobsley, M. (1980). Tests of Gastric Secretory Function. In *Scientific Foundations of Gastroenterology.* Ed. by W. Sircus and A. N. Smith. Heinemann Medical, London.

Johnston, D. (1976). Modern surgical attitudes to peptic ulceration. In *Current Surgical Practice,* vol. 1, pp. 73–113. Ed. by G. J. Hadfield and M. Hobsley. Edward Arnold, London.

Langman, M. J. S. (1979). *The Epidemiology of Chronic Digestive Disease.* Edward Arnold, London.

Rotter, J. I. and Rimoin, D. L. (1977). Peptic ulcer disease—a heterogeneous group of disorders. *Gastroenterology* **73,** 604–607.

Walsh, J. H. and Grossman, M. I. (1975). Gastrin. *New England Journal of Medicine* **292,** 1324–1332.

Wastell, C. and Lance, P. (Eds.) (1978). *Cimetidine: the Westminster Hospital Symposium, 1978.* Churchill Livingstone, Edinburgh, London and New York.

Whitfield, P. F. and Hobsley, M. (1979). A standardized technique for the performance of accurate gastric secretion studies. *Agents and Actions* **9,** 327–332.

5

Symptoms after gastric surgery

Peptic ulcer has been such a common disease, and until the very recent past has been so frequently treated by a surgical operation, that there are at present a large number of patients who have had gastroduodenal surgery. This picture is being rapidly modified by the advent of cimetidine, so that at least for the moment far fewer surgical operations designed to reduce the gastric acid secretory ability are being done. For many years, however, the problem will remain sizeable.

The nature of the operation that has been done, whether essentially a variant of vagotomy or of partial gastrectomy, makes little difference to the nature of the syndromes which may arise. This fact has only recently been realized; it was a commonly held opinion that the group of conditions called the 'dumping' syndrome (see later) were rare after vagotomy compared with their incidence after gastrectomy, but it has become apparent that dumping occurs with the same order of frequency after both types of operation. The main syndromes encountered are: recurrent peptic ulceration; dumping and allied conditions; consequences of hypochlorhydria; and mechanical problems.

Recurrent peptic ulceration

Pathogenesis

The root cause is an inadequate reduction in the ability of the stomach to secrete acid. In the case of partial gastrectomy, not enough of the body of the stomach with its parietal cells has been cut away; in the case of vagotomy, the vagal denervation of the parietal cell mass has been incomplete.

Other, less common, factors have interesting physiological bases. Failure to remove the antrum as part of a partial gastrectomy completed by a gastrojejunal anastomosis leaves the antral G cells exposed to the alkaline environment of the duodenum, and results in such massive production of gastrin as to stimulate large amounts of acid secretion from even a small gastric remnant. Some surgeons used to make a side-to-side anastomosis between the two limbs of the loop of small bowel attached to the stomach remnant as a gastrojejunostomy; this manoeuvre presumably diverted the alkaline contents of the duodenum away from the gastrojejunostomy, and there was a high incidence of recurrent ulceration on the jejunal side of the gastrojejunostomy.

Particularly interesting is the question whether recurrent ulceration after vagotomy owes anything to factors other than inadequacy of the vagotomy. An obvious possibility is that cut vagal fibres might regenerate, and this suggestion receives support from the observation that negative insulin tests shortly after the operation may become positive in later months. Another possibility is that, since the antrum is still present after vagotomy and exposed to a less acid environment than normal, hyperplasia of G cells might occur in the same way as with a retained antrum after partial gastrectomy. A few patients have been described with fasting plasma gastrin levels intermediate (200–300 pg/ml) between normal (up to 120) and Zollinger–Ellison (over 1000) levels, but the concept remains difficult to pin down.

Many investigators feel that an important cause of a *gastric* ulcer after vagotomy for duodenal ulcer is excessive reflux of alkaline and bile-containing duodenal contents into the stomach. Certainly alkaline bile can be shown to damage gastric mucosa in various experimental circumstances, but direct evidence for this thesis is lacking.

Finally, recurrent ulceration may be an expression of the Zollinger–Ellison syndrome (p. 61).

Clinical picture

The usual picture is one of recurrence of the symptoms from which the patient suffered before operation—epigastric pain relieved by food, occurring in bouts of a few days or weeks interspersed with similar or longer periods of remission. Epigastric tenderness may be elicited.

Diagnosis

Suggestive symptoms are an indication for gastroduodenoscopy, which usually confirms the diagnosis. Endoscopy may be negative unless the patient is in a period of active symptoms; in such circumstances a positive (accurate) insulin test (p. 52) makes the diagnosis highly likely. Fasting gastrin levels should be measured.

Management

If the symptoms are relieved by cimetidine, it might be reasonable to rely on long-term medical management; the patient is unlikely to be enthusiastic about operative surgery, which has already failed him once. There is as yet no experience with cimetidine treatment for more than 1 or 2 years, and in any case the symptoms are sometimes resistant to the drug; in such circumstances, recourse must be had to another operation.

After inadequate vagotomy, the surgeon usually advises a partial gastrectomy because attempting to make the vagotomy complete is likely to be technically difficult and the reported results of such attempts are not encouraging. After partial gastrectomy, assuming that the mandatory search for a retained antrum is negative, more of the body of the stomach is removed and a vagotomy added if the latter proves to be technically easy. For the Zollinger–Ellison syndrome, nothing short of *total* gastrectomy is likely to relieve the remorseless ulcer diathesis resulting from the high gastrin drive.

Recurrent ulceration may produce emergency situations such as perforation, gastric outlet obstruction, or haematemesis and melaena. The management of these situations is as for the same situations arising from primary ulceration, modified where necessary to take into account the previous operation.

Dumping and allied conditions

Several separate syndromes involving various symptoms after meals and various manifestations of nutritional deficiency have been described. They include the dumping syndrome, the late dumping syndrome, the small stomach syndrome, bilious vomiting, weight loss, disturbances of calcium metabolism, anaemia due to iron deficiency and pulmonary tuberculosis. Only recently has it been appreciated that a common physiological disturbance underlies all these conditions, at least in part, and that the key to understanding them lies in the dumping syndrome.

The dumping syndrome

The dumping syndrome was first described by Hertz (later Sir Arthur Hurst, who has been called the founder of British gastroenterology) in 1911, although the term 'dumping' was coined by Mix in 1922. It describes a large number of symptoms experienced, during a meal or during the first half hour after the meal, by patients who have been subjected to gastroduodenal operations. Not all the symptoms are necessarily encountered in every patient, but in general the symtoms fall into two groups: systemic and those related to the gastrointestinal tract.

Systemic symptoms
The patient feels faint and hot, he sweats and may have to lie down. In severe cases, the vision may grow dim and palpitations may be noted. These symptoms are similar to those of a classic vasovagal attack or simple fainting, but come on more gradually.

Gastrointestinal symptoms
The patient experiences abdominal distension and churning sensations in the epigastrium (borborygmi). The distension sometimes amounts to pain, and nausea and even vomiting may occur. The vomit often looks like pure bile, even though food has just been eaten. The most severe attacks culminate in a call to stool and the passing of a large volume (2 or more litres) of watery diarrhoea.

Associated clinical features

After partial gastrectomy, the patient often makes no complaint while in hospital, but develops symptoms when he gets home. Not every patient gets symptoms, even when specific inquiry is made. Even if the symptoms are severe, they generally improve spontaneously over the course of a year, but also if the patient is admitted to hospital for their investigation. This latter point in particular has suggested a psychogenic origin. After vagotomy, the syndrome often takes 3–6 months to develop, and longer than a year to settle down. The syndrome may follow other operations on the stomach or duodenum: simple pyloroplasty alone or (as in the case of Hertz's first patient) gastroenterostomy alone.

Foods particularly liable to produce symptoms are sweet and starchy ones, though a few patients pick out milk as a strong offender. Again, the disturbance may appear to be episodic, and since not all the symptoms may be complained of by an individual, there can be considerable doubt about the diagnosis in some patients even though many examples of the syndrome are typical and obvious. Thus there is need for a diagnostic test.

Dumping provocation test

Hypertonic glucose solution is used as the test meal: 150 ml of a 50 g/dl solution. It has been known for 25 years that such a meal reproduces the symptoms and that there is an associated rise in haematocrit. From the change of haematocrit, and on the assumption that the red cell mass does not alter, it is possible to calculate the fall in plasma volume by the equation:

$$\% \text{ fall} = 100 - \left[\frac{H_1}{100 - H_1} \times \frac{100 - H_2}{H_2} \times 100 \right]$$

where H_1 and H_2 refer to haematocrit readings before and after the glucose.

Any symptoms produced by the glucose usually settle any doubt as to whether the patient's clinical symptoms are truly dumping, and the fall in plasma volume provides an objective measurement of the physiological disturbance. In practice, patients with a fall in plasma volume of less than 8 per cent never turn out to have the syndrome, those with a fall of greater than 15 per cent are always sufferers, while patients in the intermediate range may or may not have clinical symptoms (p. 69).

Pathophysiology of dumping

The fall in circulating blood volume consequent on the contraction of the plasma volume well explains the systemic symptoms. The gastrointestinal symptoms could clearly be due to distension of the intestines. There is evidence that the presence of a hypertonic meal in the intestines draws water and electrolytes out of the whole of the extracellular compartment, with a corresponding diminution in the plasma volume. The mechanism is at least partially osmotic, because water is attracted more rapidly than the plasma electrolytes. The fall in plasma volume averages about 700 ml, but the corresponding fall in the whole of the extracellular fluid is many times greater, and this factor explains the very large volume of any diarrhoea that may result.

Since these disturbances do not arise in the normal subject, but can be produced in the normal subject by intrajejunal instillation of hypertonic glucose, it follows that the rate of delivery of a meal from the stomach into the intestines must be crucial. This would explain why all operations which can be followed by dumping have in common the factor that they destroy or bypass the pylorus. Mix's use of the term 'dumping' was meant to imply a too-rapid rate of discharge of food into the small bowel. However, measurements of the rate of gastric emptying have only recently become easy and reproducible.

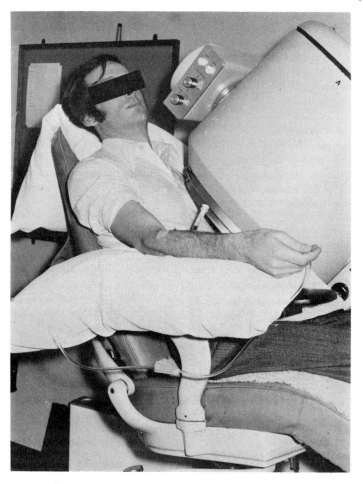

Fig. 5.1 Measurement of gastric emptying. The patient is semi-recumbent. He drinks a meal of 150 ml 50 g/dl glucose labelled with indium-112m. Gamma rays emitted by the indium are picked up by the gamma camera. The stomach region is defined, and the rate of disappearance of radioactivity from the stomach quantifies gastric emptying.

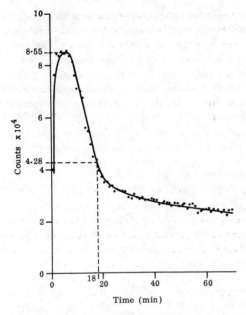

Fig. 5.2 Counts from the stomach region expressed on a linear scale and plotted against time. Convenient indices of gastric emptying are the half-life ($T_{1/2}$), the time taken for the count to decrease to half; and the percentage fall in counts during the 10 minutes following the peak. Plotting the counts on a logarithmic scale leads to a linear relationship.

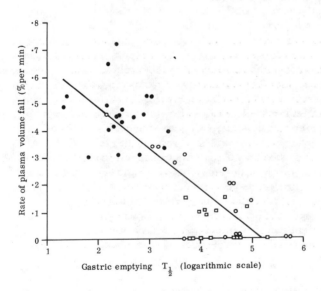

Fig. 5.3 Relationship between the percentage fall in plasma volume produced by a meal of glucose (150 ml of 50 g/dl) and the rate of emptying of the meal from the stomach. The faster the rate of emptying, the greater the fall.

Gastric emptying and dumping

The labelling of the standard hypertonic glucose meal with a radioactive marker such as indium-112m permits gastric emptying to be quantified in terms of the decay of the radioactivity in the stomach area as measured externally with a gamma camera (Fig. 5.1). The fall-off of counts with time follows a smooth curve (Fig. 5.2); if the counts are converted to their logarithms, the plot against time becomes approximately linear. Convenient representations of gastric emptying rate include the half-life of the meal in the stomach ($T_{1/2}$ min) or the percentage fall in counts during the first 10 minutes.

Dumping provocation tests performed with a radioactive-labelled meal and simultaneous measurement of gastric emptying have confirmed a close relationship between the rate of emptying and the percentage fall in plasma volume (Fig. 5.3): the faster the emptying, the greater the fall (and the greater the likelihood of symptoms). Thus there remains no reasonable doubt about the mechanism of production of symptoms. The important unanswered question is, how it is possible for two patients to have identical operative procedures and yet for one to have a normal rate of gastric emptying and the other to have a rapid rate? Also, why do patients with dumping symptoms show a tendency to spontaneous improvement? Partial answers to the second question are that rapid emptying can get slower (for unknown reasons) and that some patients adapt to the alteration in physiology and stop getting symptoms with the same fluid shift as before. There is as yet no answer to the first question.

Management

It is important to bear in mind the tendency towards spontaneous regression. Minor alterations in the patient's habits may suffice to tide him over the difficult period. He is advised to take small meals, avoiding starchy and sweet foods that are rapidly broken down to small, osmotically active, particles; to take his meals dry (ingested fluid adds to the sensation of abdominal distension); and to rest, preferably with his feet raised for a quiet ½–1 hour of relaxation after the meal. The systemic effects of lowered blood volume are relieved by rest and posture; this explains the effect on the syndrome of admission to hospital, where meals are often taken in bed and there is no question of having to report back to work immediately afterwards.

Should the symptoms be severe and persist longer than a year after the operation, the only medical treatment that has been reported to be effective is the injection of sufficient insulin, an hour before the meal, to halve the resting blood glucose concentration. The mechanism is unknown, and it is not an easy regimen to control. The only alternative is some form of surgical operation designed to reduce the rate of gastric emptying. After a vagotomy with a drainage procedure the latter can be reversed: a gastroenterostomy can be taken down or a pyloroplasty reversed to reconstitute the pylorus. After partial gastrectomy, a reversed loop of jejunum can be interposed between the stomach remnant and the rest of the small bowel. Enthusiastic early reports about the value of such procedures are difficult to assess, both because of the tendency to spontaneous resolution and because the performance of a laparotomy has a temporary non-specific effect of slowing gastric emptying. Certainly the few objective measurements which have been published before and after such operations show little permanent effect on the rate of gastric emptying except after the taking down of a gastroenterostomy.

Conditions related to dumping

Several syndromes originally dignified by separate names can now be seen to be manifestations of the dumping syndrome. Some patients find their symptoms so unpleasant that they limit their intake of food—the '*small stomach*' syndrome. The limited food intake results in *weight loss*, and, depending on the nature of the foods eaten, vitamin or calcium deficiencies may develop; with regard to the latter, both osteomalacia and osteoporosis have been described. Iron-deficiency anaemia is also common: to some degree, it is probably present in everyone by 5 years after partial gastrectomy, though similarly convincing studies are not available after vagotomy. Iron deficiency is doubtless related to the overall reduction in intake of food, but another factor is probably the hypochlorhydria produced by effective anti-ulcer surgery (next section). The overall malnutrition saps resistance, and exposes the patient to increased risk of such diseases as tuberculosis.

More controversial is the relationship between the dumping syndrome and three other conditions: bilious vomiting, postvagotomy diarrhoea and 'late dumping'.

Bilious vomiting

Particularly after a partial gastrectomy with a gastrojejunal anastomosis, the gastric emptying of the meal may be so rapid that by the time the patient feels sick the stomach fills with the contents of the duodenal loop and this liquid constitutes the vomitus. This is an undoubted cause of bilious vomiting; unfortunately, confusion may be created by the fact that a similar picture can, rarely, result from mechanical causes (p. 71).

Postvagotomy diarrhoea

A considerable mystique has grown around this variant; explosive diarrhoea is said to occur at random, and without relation to preceding meals. However, diarrhoea is also an undoubted manifestation of the severest examples of the dumping syndrome, and in the author's experience all patients with 'postvagotomy diarrhoea' have a strongly positive dumping provocation test with symptoms which culminate in diarrhoea. In some patients there may be an element of abnormal bacterial colonization of the stomach and upper small intestine (p. 150).

'Late dumping'

This name invites confusion with the dumping syndrome, and is better replaced with the phrase 'postprandial hypoglycaemia'. If, when a dumping provocation test is being performed, blood sampling is continued for 3 hours, the patient may develop systemic symptoms (tiredness, sweating, etc.) during the third hour, associated with falls in blood glucose concentration to the region of 1 mmol/l (18 mg/100 ml). The similarity of the symptoms to those produced by hypovolaemia remind one that in each case the brain cells are being starved—whether of blood or of glucose in the blood.

The mechanism producing the hypoglycaemia seems to be the excessive release of insulin in response to the rapid arrival of a carbohydrate load in the intestines and a consequently rapid absorption. Again, the common denominator with dumping is rapid gastric emptying, and the author's experience is that patients complaining of systemic symptoms 2 hours after a meal always have a positive dumping provocation test, although the reverse is not always true.

Notice that the key to diagnosis all these conditions related to dumping is the dumping provocation test.

Consequences of hypochlorhydria

The success of anti-ulcer surgery in reducing the ability of the stomach to secrete acid can have unfortunate consequences. Hypochlorhydria interferences with the absorption of iron (Sanford: *Digestive System Physiology*, Chapter 4), and so contributes to iron deficiency anaemia. Also, since hydrochloric acid helps to break up the complex molecules in which vitamin B_{12} exists in food, there is a tendency to the gradual development (after many years) of pernicious anaemia. Whether or not via the intermediary of the atrophic gastritis which often accompanies achlorhydria, carcinoma of the stomach occurs slightly, but definitely, more often in the gastric residue following partial gastrectomy than in normal stomachs. These long-term sequelae emphasize the importance of regular and prolonged follow-up of patients who have undergone anti-ulcer surgery.

Mechanical problems

Finally, and of least interest from the physiological viewpoint, various mechanical misadventures such as intussusception, volvulus of the jejunal loop and strangulation of another loop of bowel in the neighbourhood of the jejunal loop may produce indications for emergency operation. Chronic obstruction of the duodenum by kinking of the afferent loop of jejunum where it joins the stomach is a rare complication which can result in gross hypertrophy of the loop and, should it episodically release the kink, flooding of duodenal contents into the stomach remnant and a mechanical form of bilious vomiting. Mechanical problems virtually never occur after vagotomy, unless of course gastroenterostomy has been used as a drainage procedure.

Further reading

Heading, R. C. (1980). Gastric motility and emptying. In *Scientific Foundations of Gastroenterology*, pp. 287–296. Ed. by W. Sircus and A. N. Smith. Heinemann Medical, London.

Hobsley, M. (1978). Problems after gastric surgery. In *Current Surgical Practice*, vol. 2, pp. 20–38. Ed. by G. J. Hadfield and M. Hobsley. Edward Arnold, London.

Le Quesne, L. P., Hobsley, M. and Hand, B. H. (1960). The dumping syndrome. I. Factors responsible for the symptoms. *British Medical Journal* **1**, 141–147.

Lewin, M. R., Stagg, B. H. and Clark, C. G. (1973). Gastric acid secretion and diagnosis of the Zollinger–Ellison syndrome. *British Medical Journal* **2**, 139–141.

Maybury, N. K., Russell, R. C. G., Faber, R. G. and Hobsley, M. (1977). A new interpretation of the insulin test validated and then compared with the Burge test. *British Journal of Surgery* **64**, 673–676.

Thomson, J. C., Reeder, D. D., Villar, H. V. and Fender, H. R. (1975). Natural history and experience with diagnosis and treatment of the Zollinger–Ellison syndrome. *Surgery, Gynecology and Obstetrics* **140**, 721–739.

6

Liver and biliary system

The clinician's attention is directed to the liver and biliary system either by abnormal anatomy—a palpable liver—or by disturbed hepatic or biliary function. The most prominent of such disturbances of function is jaundice, but other pictures, including hepatocellular failure, ascites and portal hypertension, must be considered. Chronic upper abdominal pain as a presentation of gallstones has been discussed in Chapter 3.

Palpable liver

Many authorities state that the liver edge is often palpable in normal individuals, at least during inspiration. This cannot be true. In the normal anatomical position the inferior border of the liver lies below the costal margin (you can check this statement the next time you watch a laparotomy through an upper midline incision: the brown liver is almost always visible in the upper third of the wound), yet it cannot be felt because the liver is of softer consistency than the muscles of the overlying abdominal wall.

The liver becomes palpable because it becomes harder than normal, rather than because it becomes larger than normal. The excess tissue producing extramedullary haemopoiesis may account for the palpability of the liver in a neonate. Engorgement with blood explains the palpable liver of congestive cardiac failure, and with bile, of cholestatic (obstructive) jaundice. Alternatively, a mass or masses in the liver may be harder in consistency than the abdominal wall and so become palpable although the liver as a whole remains impalpable.

The characteristic physical signs of a palpable liver comprise a mass in the right upper quadrant of the abdomen that is not palpable in the loin (unlike the kidney which is ballotable between hands placed respectively on the loin and the anterior abdominal wall), moves downwards during inspiration and has a sharp lower border. A mass or masses in or attached to the liver have the same characteristics but no edge. If a solitary mass is rounded and lies near the tip of the right ninth costal cartilage, it is likely to be a distended gall bladder.

Liver diffusely palpable

It is usual to distinguish between smooth and nodular palpable livers: certainly the smooth mass produced by cardiac failure or acute obstructive jaundice is very different from the coarsely nodular liver of multiple metastases, but in most patients the distinction between smoothness and nodularity is insufficient to be more than a rough guide to diagnosis.

In the absence of other manifestations of hepatobiliary dysfunction, the commonest cause of a diffusely palpable liver is the presence of metastatic deposits from neoplastic disease, usually carcinomas but also reticuloses. Other causes include various forms of hepatitis and cirrhosis, and nutritional and metabolic disorders.

Solitary or multiple hepatic masses

Multiple hepatic masses nearly always turn out to be neoplastic. The same can be said of the solitary masses—one has felt the single dominant lump but other masses are present though impalpable—unless there is evidence suggesting that it is a palpable gall bladder. Rarely, a solitary mass is a primary neoplasm or chronic abscess of the liver.

Investigation and management

To know whether the hepatic involvement is diffuse or focal, and if the latter whether solitary or multiple, is an immense help in diagnosis and management. Since clinical examination is unreliable on these points, considerable attention has been paid to imaging techniques.

Imaging techniques for the liver

The longest established imaging techniques are various scintiscanning techniques after the liver has taken up a radioactive marker. Perhaps their most reliable use is in the diagnosis of a hepatic abscess: the abscess shows up on the scan as a zone of negative uptake ('cold' area) with technetium (which labels hepatocytes) but as positive uptake ('hot' area) with gallium (which labels leucocytes). The author's experience with scanning techniques for other single or multiple focal lesions has been disappointing.

The impact on this problem of newer imaging techniques such as computer assisted tomography (CAT scanning) and ultrasonography is still being assessed, but experience particularly with the latter is encouraging.

Distended gall bladder?

This possibility is investigated by ultrasound or radiologically. Plain abdominal x-rays may show gallstones. Since the gall bladder is distended but the patient is not jaundiced, the cystic duct must be blocked. An oral cholecystogram may show up the common hepatic and common bile ducts without filling the gall bladder, and these findings confirm the diagnosis of a blocked cystic duct. However, concentration of the contrast medium by the liver may not be adequate with this technique to opacify the ducts, but intravenous cholangiography is usually successful.

A gall bladder palpable due to chronic distension is an indication for cholecystectomy: the distending contents trapped in the gall bladder will be found to be either mucus (*mucocele*) or pus (*empyema of the gall bladder*).

Secondary carcinoma?

The liver is one of the most common sites (with the lungs) for secondary carcinomatous deposits. The commonest sites of the primary lesions are the stomach, colon and pancreas. If there are no physical symptoms or signs to establish a preferential order, the colon should be investigated by simoidoscopy and barium enema before the stomach by gastroduodenoscopy and barium meal. This is because barium introduced proximal to an incomplete colonic obstruction may become inspissated and convert the obstruction into a complete one. Carcinoma of the pancreas is discussed elsewhere (p. 41).

Breast and bronchial carcinomas also commonly metastasize to the liver. The foregoing paragraph assumes that there is no clinical evidence of carcinoma of these sites, and that the chest x-ray is negative.

Reticulosis?

If there are no suggestive clinical features such as a palpable spleen or lymph nodes, and if the blood count and chest x-ray are normal, a reticulosis is unlikely.

Tissue diagnosis

If all the previous lines of investigation draw a blank, it is unlikely that further progress towards the correct diagnosis will be achieved without obtaining a specimen of the liver for histological examination. The first line of attack is *needle-biopsy*: in expert hands this is remarkably safe, but there is always the possibility of severe haemorrhage from an organ as vascular as the liver. The patient is therefore admitted to hospital, 2 units of blood are cross-matched and the prothrombin time is checked. The liver is the main site of protein synthesis in the body, and therefore the main source of most of the blood clotting factors. The problem is further discussed on p. 83, but if the prothrombin time is abnormally prolonged or the patient is jaundiced, vitamin K_1 10 mg IM should be given daily for 3 days before the needle-biopsy.

The usual route is across the costodiaphragmatic recess of the pleural cavity and through the diaphragm, the needle piercing the eighth, ninth or tenth intercostal space in the mid-axillary line. However, if the liver is clearly palpable in the right upper quadrant, the subcostal route in the mid-clavicular line can be used. A solitary lesion can be directly aimed at, but one important contraindication to needle-biopsy must be remembered: the possibility that the mass is a hydatid cyst. Needling a hydatid cyst can disseminate the disease throughout the peritoneal cavity or produce immediate death from anaphylaxis.

Other ways of obtaining a tissue diagnosis, via peritoneoscopy or formal laparotomy, may need to be considered.

Three important examples of lesions which may present as a soliary mass in the liver are presented below.

Hydatid disease (echinococcosis)

The *Echinococcus* is a minute worm which inhabits the small intestine of dogs and their wild relatives such as foxes. The eggs are passed in the faeces and eaten by sheep and cattle; embryos hatch from the eggs in the duodenum and penetrate through the intestinal wall to gain the circulation, and widespread dissemination follows. Dogs become reinfected by eating the carcasses of animals that have died of the disease

Man becomes infected if he allows his food to become contaminated with canine faeces. The condition is common wherever sheep and cattle are associated with dogs; for example, Australasia, the Argentine and South Wales. The larval stage or hydatid cysts can lodge in any tissue or region of the body. Their presence may be detected at an early stage by interference with important and sensitive functions (e.g. in the eye or the brain), but otherwise the condition remains silent for many years until the size of the lesion attracts attention or leakage of liquid through the cyst wall produces an allergic reaction or eosinophilia. The liver is the most common site, and traumatic rupture of a large hepatic hydatid cyst can produce sudden death from anaphylaxis.

The *diagnosis* is made by immunological tests such as the complement fixation test or an intradermal injection of antigen prepared from sterile cyst fluid.

Treatment is mechanical: the surgeon exposes the outer surface of the cyst, takes every possible precaution against local contamination by spillage, aspirates as much as possible of the cyst liquid and replaces it with 10 per cent formaldehyde solution to sterilize the germinative layer of the cyst wall, and then enucleates the whole cyst.

Amoebic liver abscess

Intestinal amoebiasis in general is considered in Chapter 8. However, *Entamoeba histolytica* secretes a cytotoxin which destroys the intestinal mucosa, and the parasite thereby gains access to the blood stream and is carried to the liver. Here it produces usually solitary, though sometimes multiple, inflammatory lesions which progress to necrosis. The resulting abscess contains soft, chocolate-brown material.

The clinical picture is usually a sudden onset of rigors and prostration, but sometimes there is an insidiously increasing pain in the right hypochrondrium. In either case, leucocytosis, a raised diaphragm on chest x-ray and a pleural rub are common.

The diagnosis is confirmed by examining the stools for cysts, ova and parasites.

Treatment is in general medical, the modern drug of choice being metronidazole (Flagyl) although emetine hydrochloride can be given if metronidazole fails; sometimes it is necessary to combine medical treatment with needle-aspiration of the abscess.

Primary hepatic tumours

There are two main histological varieties of hepatoma—hepatocellular carcinoma and cholangiocarcinoma—and a mixed type, together with the hepatoblastoma of infancy.

Primary carcinoma of the liver, though much less common than secondary carcinoma, has an interestingly high incidence in certain geographical areas such as among the Bantu tribe of southern Africa and the Chinese. It is not clear whether the aetiological factor is dietary, racial or some other geographically linked agent. For example, aflatoxin, a substance highly carcinogenic in animals, is produced by a mould which frequently contaminates groundnuts and cereals stored in tropical conditions. Leaving aside these high incidence areas, the most important predisposing factor appears to be multinodular cirrhosis, and in such circumstances the carcinoma is often multifocal from its inception. Hepatomas also sometimes occur in patients with other diseases affecting the liver; for example, viral hepatitis, biliary cirrhosis secondary to atresia of the bile ducts and galactosaemia. Alpha$_1$-fetoprotein is often found in the serum. This globulin is a normal component of the plasma proteins of human fetuses, but disappears from the circulation a few weeks after birth. Its subsequent reappearance is a good marker for primary liver cancer.

The condition has a grave prognosis: widespread metastases tend to develop at a relatively early stage. However, a few patients have been saved by formal (i.e. with prior control of the regional blood vessels and bile ducts) resections of the liver, usually a right or left hemihepatectomy; hepatic transplantation has been tried but the results have been disappointing.

Jaundice

Jaundice is a yellow discoloration of skin and mucous membranes due to an excess accumulation of bilirubin in the tissues. The associated plasma concentration of bilirubin exceeds 18 μmol/l (1 mg/100 ml).

At least in adults (for paediatric jaundice, see p. 89) it is possible clearly to distinguish two types of jaundice, characterized respectively by an excess of unconjugated or of conjugated bilirubin (Sanford: *Digestive System Physiology*, Chapter 4). Bilirubin is produced in the reticuloendothelial system, particularly the spleen, from the haemoglobin of old erythrocytes. It is only very slightly soluble in water in its unconjugated form, but is transported to the liver in the circulation bound to the plasma albumin, and into the hepatocytes after transfer of the binding to two other proteins designated ligandin (or Y) and Z. Within the hepatocyte, bilirubin is conjugated with glucuronic acid to form the diglucuronide; this conjugated bilirubin is soluble in water. The reaction of conjugation is catalysed by an enzyme, bilirubin UDP-glucuronyl transferase. The conjugated bilirubin is excreted into the bile canaliculi and thence via the main bile ducts into the duodenum.

In the small intestine the conjugation is broken down by bacterial enzymes, the unconjugated bilirubin is reduced to colourless urobilinogen, and some of this is reabsorbed but the remainder is excreted in the faeces. The reabsorbed urobilinogen is partly re-excreted by the liver, but the rest appears in the urine. Thus urine normally contains some urobilinogen but no (insoluble) bilirubin, while faeces contains some urobilinogen (stercobilinogen). These statements form the key to the difference between the two main types of jaundice.

When unconjugated bilirubin accumulates because of some fault on the pathway between the spleen and the hepatocytes, there is no bile in the urine and the jaundice is called *acholuric*. However, an accumulation of conjugated bilirubin due to obstruction to the excretory pathway beyond the hepatocyte results in the regurgitation of conjugated soluble bilirubin back into the plasma and its consequent appearance in the urine. This type of jaundice is called *cholestatic* or *obstructive*; if the obstruction is complete, urobilinogen disappears from the urine and faeces because no bilirubin is reaching the intestine to become urobilinogen. Stercobilin, the brown pigment produced normally in the faeces from urobilinogen, is thus absent from the faeces in obstructive jaundice: the stools become clay-coloured.

Acholuric jaundice

Unconjugated bilirubin accumulates in the blood either because of an excess formation from haemoglobin (i.e. excessive haemolysis) or because of disturbances of uptake into the liver cell or of conjugation. The non-haemolytic group are familial.

Haemolytic jaundice

Both stool and urine are normal in colour and there is no pruritus—the latter is an important distinction from cholestatic jaundice. Depending on the balance between haemolysis and the regeneration of erythrocytes, there may be a significant anaemia. The jaundice is mild and of a lemon yellow colour; it never takes on the green tinge of advanced cholestasis.

The spleen is palpable in chronic forms, and ulcers occur in the region of the ankles in some types (the cause for the latter is not clear). Gallstones of pigment type are common (p. 22).

The plasma unconjugated bilirubin levels are only moderately raised (18–90 μmol/l, 1–5 mg/100 ml), and free haemoglobin may be detectable. The reticulocyte count of the blood is increased in proportion to the rate of regeneration of red cells; in appropriate cases increased fragility of the red cells can be demonstrated, the survival of ^{51}Cr-labelled red cells is reduced and their uptake by the spleen increased.

Hepatic needle-biopsy may be necessary to distinguish some patients with Gilbert's disease (p. 79) who have a minor reduction in the life span of their erythrocytes: in haemolytic anaemia the liver is packed with iron (as may other tissues as well—tissue siderosis; Sanford: *Digestive System Physiology*, Chapter 4).

Excessive haemolysis may be due to abnormalities of the erythrocyte or to extracorpuscular causes.

Abnormalities of the erythrocytes include the increased osmotic fragility of the rounded red cells of *congenital spherocytosis*, deficiencies of various enzymes within the cells concerned with carbohydrate metabolism (e.g. glucose-6-phosphate dehydrogenase) and abnormal haemoglobins. In *sickle-cell disease* the abnormal haemoglobin is called haemoglobin S; it crystallizes when oxygen tension is reduced, resulting in a severe crisis of blood destruction accompanied by abdominal or peripheral pain. The disease is common in Arabs and Negroes. A particularly common risk of relative hypoxia occurs in the induction of anaesthesia, and the appropriate screening test must be performed before administering an anaesthetic to patients from the high-risk groups. A similar condition, *thalassaemia*—common in individuals from the Mediterranean seaboard—is due to failure to produce beta chains. Other abnormal haemoglobins have been described in various ethnic groups.

An unknown abnormality of the red cells is responsible in a few individuals for an excessive sensitivity to the acid pH that may occur during sleep—*paroxysmal nocturnal haemoglobinuria.*

Extracorpuscular causes include *severe infections* (malaria, septicaemia, viral pneumonia), *incompatible blood transfusion, burns* (the red cells are damaged by exposure to heat), *drugs* such as phenacetin, *haemolytic disease of the newborn* (p. 90 and *acquired haemolytic anaemia.* The latter may be *secondary* to other diseases, particularly of the reticuloendothelial system, such as Hodgkin's disease and leukaemia, but also uraemia and carcinomatosis; or *idiopathic*, due to autoimmunization, in which case the Coombs' test (p. 90) is positive.

Non-haemolytic familial jaundice

The commonest variety is *Gilbert's syndrome.* This condition is inherited as an autosomal dominant, the patients being heterozygous for a single mutant gene. It is usually mild, and the jaundice so inconspicuous most of the time that the condition may only be diagnosed at a routine medical examination. However, the icterus may deepen following any intercurrent infection, or after starvation: a 400-calorie (16.8 mJ) diet for 24 hours has been used as a diagnostic test. Episodes of deeper jaundice may be associated with mild nausea and discomfort in the hepatic region, but usually there are no symptoms and the prognosis is excellent. The total plasma bilirubin concentration rarely exceeds 54 μmol/l (3 mg/100 ml); the hepatic histology determined by liver biopsy is normal and there is no other evidence of hepatic dysfunction. The cause is probably a disturbance of uptake by the liver cells combined with some reduction in the UDP-glucuronyl transferase, but it is interesting that some patients have a slight reduction in the life span of their erythrocytes and this can cause confusion with the haemolytic anaemias (p. 78).

Other varieties are very rare: they include the *Crigler–Najjar* type in which there seems to be a complete absence of the transferase and affected babies usually die within the first year.

These conditions show a considerable overlap with varieties of familial jaundice in which conjugated rather than non-conjugated pigment accumulates; for example, the *Rotor* and *Dubin–Johnson* types.

Cholestatic jaundice

The dark urine, pale stools and high concentration of conjugated bilirubin in the plasma make the overall diagnosis of cholestatic jaundice easy. In long-standing or severe cases, the green colour of the jaundice and the presence of itching are also characteristic, as is the rise in plasma alkaline phosphatase concentration. The normal range of the latter is 3–13 King–Armstrong or 21–85 international units per decilitre, and the increase in obstructive jaundice does not seem to be due to the failure of excretion of the enzyme via the bile into the intestine but to increased production in the hepatocytes. Other isoenzymes are secreted by the intestines and by bone; to determine whether an increase in plasma alkaline phosphatase originates in the liver, the simplest test is to measure plasma 5-nucleotidase concentration which rises only in hepatobiliary disturbance.

The crucial subdivision of cholestatic jaundice, since it distinguishes those who need a surgical operation from those who do not, is into *extrahepatic* and *intrahepatic* obstruction. The direct distinction between these two categories has recently become much easier with the help of three special techniques: ultrasonography, endoscopic retrograde cholangiopancreatography (ERCP) and percutaneous transhepatic cholangiography (PTC).

Endoscopic retrograde cholangiopancreatography (ERCP)
The technique of cannulating the common bile duct with a tube passed via a duodenoscope in a sedated patient is now well established, and the success rate in experienced hands is of the order of 90 per cent. Injection of a radio-opaque contrast medium along the tube outlines the biliary passages from below, up to the level of any mechanical block (Fig. 6.1). Thus the decision whether the lower border of the block is in the common bile or hepatic ducts, and therefore possibly amenable to surgical intervention, or else in the smaller hepatic bile duct radicles or even at hepatocellular level, can readily be made (p. 86). Perhaps of even greater technical importance to the surgeion is the *upper* level of the block, and that is best shown by PTC.

Percutaneous transhepatic cholangiography (PTC)
The percutaneous passage of a needle into the liver for the introduction of radio-opaque contrast material into the dilated biliary passages above a block has been used for many years. Only recently, however, has a modification of this technique been developed using a very fine flexible needle, which makes the method safer by reducing the risk that inadvertent movements of respiration by the patient might result in hepatic damage and consequent haemorrhage.

If gross distension of the biliary tree, of the type produced by extrahepatic or 'surgical' obstruction, is present, manipulating the needle to enter an intrahepatic bile duct is usually possible, and the injected contrast produces

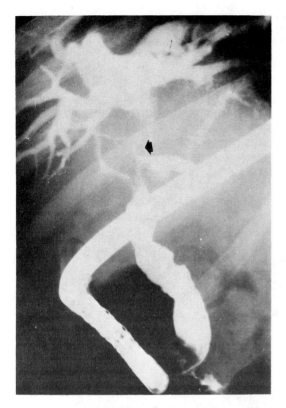

Fig. 6.1 X-ray obtained by ERCP. An endoscope has been passed into the second part of the duodenum and used to cannulate the common bile duct via the papilla of Vater. Injected contrast material has filled the biliary system and demonstrated a long stricture (arrow) just below the confluence of left and right hepatic ducts. Sometimes the blockage produced by the stricture is more complete, no contrast passes the stricture and its upper end can then not be visualized by this technique. PTC is useful in such cases (see Fig. 6.2).

excellent definition of the site of the obstruction (Fig. 6.2a). It is even possible by this route to dilate a stricture and insert an endoprosthesis (Fig. 6.2b).

Leakage of bile into the peritoneal cavity and a resultant generalized peritonitis is always a possibility after this investigation, and may require urgent laparotomy. Precautions against haemorrhage are as for before hepatic needle-biopsy. Cholangitis due to the introduction of pathogenic organisms into a still-obstructed system is another and a very serious complication.

Extrahepatic ('surgical') cholestatic jaundice
Provided that no previous cholecystectomy has been performed, the presence or absence of a dilated, palpable gall bladder distinguishes between patients in whom the obstruction is distal or proximal to the point at which the cystic duct joins the common hepatic duct to form the common bile duct. The causes of

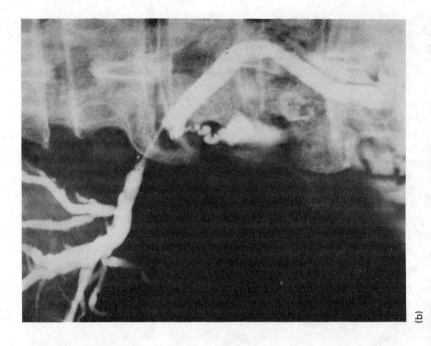

(a)

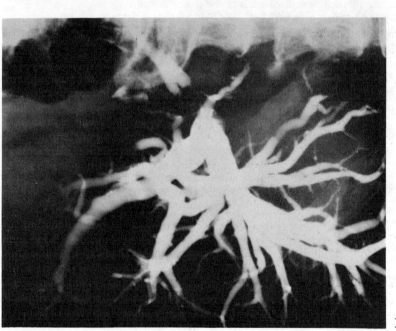

(b)

Fig. 6.2 Percutaneous transhepatic cholangiography (PTC), diagnostic and sometimes therapeutic. (a) A fine flexible needle has been inserted into the hepatic duct system, dilated proximal to a block just below the confluence of the right and left hepatic ducts. (b) The stricture producing the obstruction has been negotiated and a prosthesis inserted, all by the transhepatic route, and contrast now enters the common bile duct. (Films kindly provided by Dr. Richard Mason)

obstruction are luminal (gallstones; or parasites such as the liver fluke that is so common in South-east Asia); strictures of the wall, whether benign (traumatic), inflammatory or neoplastic (cholangiocarcinoma); or extrinsic pressure from disease of neighbouring structures such as enlarged lymph nodes of reticuloses or secondary carcinomatosis, or primary carcinoma of the head of the pancreas.

The technique of ERCP provides a means of dealing with some types of intraluminal obstruction, at least with one or a few gallstones up to about 2.5 cm in diameter. The endoscopist with special training can perform a diathermy-sphincterotomy of the duodenal opening of the common bile duct, and can pass instruments such as wire baskets up the duct to engage the stones and manipulate them into the duodenum. Such skill is not available yet in many centres, and in any case, since the stones have originated in a diseased gall bladder which is likely to make more stones, the logical treatment is to remove the gall bladder and this requires laparotomy. Thus, except in the special case that the patient has already undergone cholecystectomy (or there is a strong contraindication to general anaesthesia), laparotomy is usually required.

Before laparotomy, attention must be paid to the derangements of physiology produced by obstructive jaundice. Anaemia is common; it is due to an increased bleeding tendency in association with a reduction in hepatic blood-clotting factors, with thrombocytopenia and with a shortened life span of the erythrocytes (so that unconjugated bilirubin also may increase in concentration in the plasma of patients with long-standing jaundice). The liver is the main site in which synthesis of proteins is performed, and is concerned with the production of most of the factors involved in the coagulation of the blood; prolonged cholestasis can result in deficiency of factors VII, II and X, later of IX and ultimately even of V and I (fibrinogen). Vitamin K is needed for the production within the liver of factors II, VII, IX and X, and because the vitamin is fat-soluble and cannot be absorbed from the small intestine in the absence of bile, its deficiency is particularly likely in patients with cholestatic jaundice. The overall defect is revealed by prolongation of the one-stage prothrombin time test, but even if a normal result is obtained the patient should receive vitamin K_1 by intramuscular injection, 10 mg daily for 3 days. If this measure fails to restore the prothrombin time to normal, the transfusion of fresh whole blood, or of concentrates of the particular factors found to be deficient by more refined tests, is necessary.

Obstruction to the extrahepatic biliary tree, particularly if due to a foreign body such as a gallstone, is commonly associated with infectious processes such as ascending cholangitis or septicaemia. Any suspicion of these conditions (pyrexia, rigors, severe constitutional disturbance including headache and delirium) demand broad-spectrum antibiotics.

Jaundiced patients are also prone to acute renal failure (the so-called hepatorenal syndrome) if the plasma bilirubin concentration exceeds 170 μmol/l (10 mg/100 ml). Maintenance of a rapid production of urine during and for 24 hours after operation with the osmotic diuretic, mannitol, has been shown to reduce the incidence of this complication. The mechanism whereby jaundice damages the renal tubules is unknown.

Principles of laparotomy
The extrahepatic site of obstruction is to be identified, its nature determined and the obstruction either removed or bypassed so that bile can once again drain from the liver into the small intestine: prolonged complete biliary obstruction is incompatible with life.

Sometimes an exact diagnosis has been made before operation, by PTC or ERCP; even in such cases it is often advisable to obtain an up-to-date picture of the biliary tree by peroperative cholangiography (p. 32).

Calculi in the common bile duct are removed with the aid of instruments introduced into the duct, either via a hole made in the supraduodenal portion of the duct or via the papilla of Vater after opening the second part of the duodenum and slitting open the papilla so as to improve access to the intramural portion of the duct. Occasionally it is necessary to use a combined approach in order to deal with a large stone impacted in the narrow terminal segment of the common duct. All stones are removed and any sludge or mud washed through into the duodenum until the operator is confident that the duct is clear. After supraduodenal exploration the hole in the common bile duct is only partially closed, around a T-tube (see Fig. 3.8). See Chapter 3 for further details of management.

The other major group of causes of obstruction at the lower end of the common bile duct is a *tumour*—either a cholangiocarcinoma arising from the mucous membrane of the bile duct itself or a carcinomatous mass in the neighbouring head of the pancreas.

Very occasionally the obstruction may be an expression of chronic pancreatitis. Because of this possibility (and indeed a stone impacted at the lower end of the duct, or even a duodenal ulcer of the second part of the duodenum, can feel just like a carcinoma of the head of the pancreas), it is important to have histological confirmation of the nature of the lesion so the second part of the duodenum may have to be opened to permit biopsy. If carcinoma is confirmed, a curative procedure may be attempted—*pancreato-duodenectomy* or *Whipple's operation*. The head of the pancreas up to the right border of the portal vein is removed with the contiguous gastric antrum and the first, second and third parts of the duodenum (Fig. 3.12a, b). This is a major procedure with a high operative mortality. In the absence of obvious signs of secondary spread, there is a reasonable chance of a good prognosis with bile duct carcinoma because such a lesion is likely to produce jaundice at an early stage; with carcinoma of the head of the pancreas, however, many surgeons feel that the operation is not justifiable and simply bypass the obstruction (e.g. cholecystenterostomy and, usually, since gastric outlet obstruction impends, gastroenterostomy as well—Fig. 3.12c).

In the case of the foregoing conditions, the gall bladder (if present) will have been found to be distended. If the gall bladder is empty—a much less common finding—the obstruction must be sought in the right and left hepatic or the common hepatic duct. Peroperative cholangiography shows a normal duct system (in which case the jaundice is due to disease at the hepatocellular level and laparotomy has turned out to be unnecessary), or a localized stricture, or a pattern of several areas of ragged strictures with intervening dilatations. Very occasionally a filling defect due to a stone is found and dealt with by exploration.

A localized stricture is usually due to previous surgical trauma (e.g. during a previous cholecystectomy) but sometimes is due to an intrinsic cholangio-carcinoma or to extrinsic pressure from masses such as enlarged lymph nodes in the porta hepatis. The principles of management are again biopsy to establish the diagnosis, and excision with reconstruction of the bile duct or else bypass of the obstruction. These operations are technically difficult and best left to a surgeon with special experience in this field.

Multiple irregularities of the bile ducts may be due to *primary biliary cirrhosis* (p. 87), cholangiocarcinoma, or the group of conditions including pericholangitis and sclerosing cholangitis. The latter two conditions are a complication of chronic inflammatory disease of the bowel (often Crohn's disease or ulcerative colitis; see Chapter 8).

Extrahepatic or intrahepatic?

The preceding description of extrahepatic cholestasis has assumed that a correct diagnosis that the condition is present has been achieved by ultrasonography, PTC or ERCP and therefore laparotomy has been undertaken. This assumption begs the question of how the clinician reached the position of deciding to perform PTC or ERCP. These two investigations require considerable skill which is not available in every centre, and, particularly in the case of PTC, entail some risk. Therefore they are not undertaken unless the clinical evidence points clearly towards a surgical cause of the jaundice. On the other hand, unless the clinical evidence points unequivocally to a 'medical' intrahepatic cause, one must bear in mind that the longer the patient remains jaundiced, the more likely are serious complications of the group collectively called liver failure (p. 92) and the greater the risk of subsequent laparotomy. It is a tragedy if the post-mortem examination of a patient who has died from jaundice and consequent liver failure reveals an extrahepatic obstructive cause that could easily have been relieved by a surgical procedure. Yet the risks of an unnecessary anaesthetic and laparotomy in a patient whose liver is damaged are also considerable. This is the essential conundrum which makes every patient with cholestatic jaundice a challenge to the clinician.

In the past, considerable reliance has been placed on tests of hepatocellular function such as plasma transaminase and albumin concentration and on the concentration of plasma alkaline phosphatase. The rise in the latter (p. 80) is proportional to the completeness of obstruction and therefore very high levels (above 200 i.u./l) are likely to signify the complete obstruction which is probably due to mechanical obstruction of the larger bile passages and therefore amenable to surgery. Lesser rises, in the range 85–150 i.u./l, are more likely to result from the incomplete obstruction caused by damage at hepatocellular level. The transaminases (aspartate aminotransferase and alanine aminotransferase) leak out from damaged hepatocytes and so a rise in the plasma concentration above the normal range (50–150 i.u./l for both) is likely to represent a hepatocellular cause for the jaundice. The hepatocytes manufacture albumin, and so damage to hepatocytes is likely to result in a fall in the concentration of albumin in the plasma. Remember that the normal turnover rate of plasma albumin is 3 g per day and that it is vital for preserving the oncotic pressure of the plasma (Sanford: *Digestive System Physiology*, Chapter 4).

While in general the above statements hold good, they are unreliable in the context of the individual patient: hepatocellular damage can produce *complete* cholestasis and long-standing cholestasis can produce hepatocellular damage.

Bearing in mind that PTC and ERCP are not available everywhere, that non-invasive imaging techniques such as ultrasonography are never contraindicated and give useful evidence in patients with gross anatomical changes such as gallstones or carcinoma of the head of the pancreas or grossly dilated biliary passages, and that strong clinical evidence pointing towards any individual disease must be taken into consideration, three rules of guidance can be stated.

1. *Complete obstruction lasting for a week requires laparotomy.* Completeness of the obstruction can be diagnosed by the absence of urobilinogen from every sample of urine. The diagnosis is probably a malignant obstruction to the bile duct because the jaundice due to gallstones is often intermittent since the obstructing stone is likely to work free from time to time.

2. *Coexisting constitutional disturbance or an intra-abdominal palpable mass requires laparotomy.* Constitutional disturbance (fever, rigors, sweating, prostration) indicates one or a combination of ascending cholangitis, septicaemia and liver abscess. In half the cases there is a primary focus of infection elsewhere in the abdomen (e.g. acute appendicitis) and if there is evidence of such a focus it must be dealt with urgently. Cultures of samples of blood are set up and, in the absence of obvious sources of infection, alternative diagnoses such as infectious mononucleosis, malaria, Weil's disease, syphilis, tuberculosis and yellow fever are considered and the appropriate investigations done. If the palpable mass is a gall bladder, Courvoisier's law states that in a patient with jaundice a palpable gall bladder suggests that the obstruction is not due to gallstones. This is because if the obstruction is due to a gallstone, the latter originated in the gall bladder which has therefore been the seat of chronic inflammation and consequently fibrosed and indistensible. If the palpable mass is elsewhere in the abdomen, it is probably a carcinoma which has given rise to secondary deposits in lymph nodes in the porta hepatis. In either case, early laparotomy is indicated.

3. *Long-standing jaundice requires laparotomy, or at least PTC or ERCP.* This rule applies even if there is some evidence that points towards intrahepatic cholestasis. PTC or ERCP should be performed after a week has passed; if they are not available, laparotomy should not be deferred longer than 6 weeks after the onset.

Intrahepatic ('medical') cholestatic jaundice
This section details the more important conditions producing jaundice by interfering with the excretion of conjugated bilirubin either at hepatocellular

level or in the small intrahepatic bile canaliculi and collecting ducts. Many of
these conditions do not necessarily produce jaundice, and inasmuch as they
can produce a palpable liver without jaundice, they are also the possible
diagnoses of a diffusely enlarged, otherwise symptomless, palpable liver
(p. 74).

Primary biliary cirrhosis   This is an interesting condition since its site of
obstruction may be both extrahepatic (p. 81) and in the liver itself where it
narrows the small bile ducts. Most patients are middle-aged women and the
onset is insidious, with pruritus often preceding jaundice by some months.
Skin xanthomas (yellow tumours) are common, as are diarrhoea, steatorrhoea
and weight loss; bleeding from duodenal ulceration (the cause of this
association is unknown) is a frequent complication, and in the later stages
portal hypertension develops with a risk of bleeding from oesophageal varices.
Collagen diseases such as rheumatoid arthritis, scleroderma and Sjögren's
syndrome may accompany the condition, and most patients with the disease
can be shown to have immunological abnormalities of which the typical
finding is a positive mitochondrial antibody test. Needle- (or open) biopsy of
the liver clinches the diagnosis: the histology is that of a chronic, non-
suppurative, destructive cholangitis. The condition progresses relentlessly to
death, but the rate of deterioration can be very slow.

Viral hepatitis   There are several forms of this condition, the best characterized
being virus A hepatitis and virus B hepatitis. The virus A type affects
particularly children and young adults, is transmitted usually by the
faecal–oral route although the blood is also infectious, and has an incubation
period of 15–20 days. Type B hepatitis has a longer incubation period of
50–160 days, transmission is usually by the parenteral or venereal routes and
the typical mechanism is the transfusion of blood of blood products, although
semen, faeces and urine are also infectious. Most patients with type B hepatitis
can be shown to possess a particular antigen which was first encountered in an
Australian aborigine and was therefore called Australia antigen. It is now
called hepatitis B antigen or HBAg; in the average case it has disappeared
from the serum in about 4 weeks from the onset of symptoms but it may
persist as a chronic carrier state.

The clinical course of type A hepatitis is, on average, milder than that of
type B; in patients in whom jaundice develops, mortality figures of about 0.1
per cent are quoted for type A but as high as 12 per cent in some series of type
B. In both types, the course can be extremely variable, ranging from a
subclinical infection which manifests itself by a chance finding of an increase
in plasma transaminase levels (and HBAg in type B), through an anicteric
clinical illness of malaise, gastrointestinal and influenza-like symptoms, to the
complete picture with jaundice. A prodromal period of days (or even 2 weeks)
of malaise and other non-specific symptoms, particularly anorexia, precedes
icterus, of which the first sign is darkening of the urine due to bilirubinuria.
Once jaundice appears, the patient usually feels better though the liver is often
palpable and tender and itching may arise.

In jaundiced patients the disease usually lasts about 3 weeks before gradual
recovery. Sometimes cholestasis continues for several weeks and the possibility
of the jaundice being 'surgical' has to be considered; needle-biopsy is helpful
in preventing an unnecessary laparotomy. The histology of both types is

identical: an acute inflammatory process involves the whole liver although necrosis is most obvious in the centre of the lobule and the reactive infiltration with leucocytes and histiocytes is most marked near the portal tracts. A severe form of the disease is fulminant hepatitis which produces acute hepatocellular failure and kills the patient in 10 days.

There is no specific treatment for viral hepatitis, although corticosteroids can depress the serum bilirubin concentration without affecting the extent of hepatic necrosis. A low fat, low protein, high carbohydrate diet is traditional, but probably the best diet is whatever the patient finds appetizing. For the treatment of a patient with severe hepatocellular failure, see p. 95.

Following recovery from jaundice there is a variable period of depression, fatiguability, anorexia, alcohol intolerance, and pain and tenderness in the region of the liver—the posthepatitis syndrome. In the end recovery is usually complete, but in about 5 per cent of cases there follows one or more relapses and a few patients progress to chronic hepatitis (below) and cirrhosis (p. 89).

In the case of type A hepatitis, immune serum globulin (ISG) from patients who have had the disease confers some protection if given before or within 2 weeks of exposure, to individuals at risk; for example, to close household contacts of a patient, hospital workers accidentally contaminated with blood from a patient with the condition, or travellers in the tropics—especially if they propose to diverge from the beaten track of the major tourist routes. The value of ISG in type B disease is not certain.

The question of whether the chronic HBAg carrier is dangerous as a source of infection remains unresolved.

Drug jaundice   Drugs can produce jaundice by interfering with the metabolism of bilirubin in all its stages from its formation in the reticuloendothelial system to its appearance in the major bile ducts. The two most common causes of cholestatic jaundice amongst the drugs are testosterone, which seems to act at the level of the microscopic collecting tubules, and chlorpromazine, which causes cellular proliferation in the small intrahepatic bile duct radicles. When extrahepatic obstruction has been eliminated, a history of ingestion of these drugs can usually be accepted as diagnostic; confirmation can, however, be obtained by histological examination of a hepatic needle-biopsy. Oestrogens, as in the contraceptive pill, can produce cholestatic jaundice, but, in relation to the vast numbers of women taking the treatment, the incidence of this complication is very small.

There is a long list of other drugs which can produce jaundice. Some are directly toxic to the liver cells, and, like carbon tetrachloride, can result in acute hepatic failure (p. 95). Damage can even be produced by such commonly used remedies as salicylates and paracetamol. Another group appear to produce a hypersensitivity reaction; the volatile anaesthetic agent halothane is an example, and if this agent has been used in a first operation on a patient but a second has become necessary during the same hospital admission, the anaesthetist avoids using halothane the second time because the patient may have been sensitized by the first exposure.

Chronic hepatitis   This condition is defined as chronic liver disease that has existed for longer than 6 months. Hepatic tissue obtained by needle-biopsy usually permits differentiation into two distinct histological groups. In *chronic persistent hepatitis* there is a periportal cellular infiltrate and not much necrosis or fibrosis: the prognosis is good. The most common aetiological factor is an attack of virus hepatitis type A or type B, but other precipitating stresses include long-standing ulcerative colitis or Crohn's disease, schistosomiasis or acute alcoholic hepatitis. In *chronic active hepatitis* there is the same periportal inflammation but this extends into the parenchyma and is associated with piecemeal necrosis and the formation of septa between groups of liver cells. This condition has a much more serious prognosis as most cases are irreversible and progress to hepatic cirrhosis. While virus hepatitis (usually type B, but also possibly type A) is one of the aetiological factors, the most common form of initiating attack is an HBAg-negative form of hepatitis which is sometimes called active chronic 'lupoid' hepatitis. This is predominantly a disease of young (10- to 25-year-old) females, is usually associated with immunological changes such as a positive lupus erythematosus (LE) cell phenomenon, antinuclear factor and smooth muscle antibody, may involve other organs such as the thyroid (in the form of Hashimoto's autoimmune thyroiditis), and may respond favourably (though not permanently) to treatment with corticosteroids. Other causes of chronic active hepatitis include acute alcoholic liver disease, other drugs (e.g. methyldopa), viral infections of childhood such as rubella, Wilson's disease (p. 93) and alpha$_1$-antitrypsin deficiency (p. 91).

Hepatic cirrhosis This condition is defined as the combination of fibrosis spread widely throughout the liver (although not necessarily affecting every liver lobule) together with the formation of nodules. The fibrosis follows necrosis, and the nodules represent attempted regeneration of liver tissue. The naked eye appearances of the liver depend on the strength of the regeneration: vigorous regeneration results in large nodules (macronodular cirrhosis), poor regeneration in small nodules (about 1 cm, micronodular), while a mixed form also occurs. Cirrhosis may be preceded by chronic active hepatitis, and so all the aetiological factors mentioned above under that heading apply to cirrhosis. One must add prolonged cholestasis, prolonged hepatic venous engorgement due to right heart failure or occlusion of the hepatic veins, schistosomiasis, congenital syphilis, some rare conditions such as galactosaemia, glycogen storage disease and certain drugs. After all such possibilities have been excluded, there remains a considerable residue (about 40 per cent in the United Kingdom, less in countries where alcoholism is more prevalent) of patients in whom the origin of the cirrhosis is unknown; these cases are usually labelled *cryptogenic cirrhosis*.

Neonatal jaundice

There are good reasons for separating the discussion of jaundice in infants from that in adults. First, many of the rarer conditions producing neonatal jaundice are incompatible with prolonged life and therefore are never encountered in the adult. Secondly, the distinction between haemolytic and cholestatic jaundice is less clear-cut so that, for example, haemolysis can give rise to bile in the urine. Thirdly, the so-called 'physiological' jaundice due to immaturity of the hepatocytes is very common at birth but then resolves in the next 2 or 3 weeks, and this condition is only seen in the neonatal period.

The management of neonatal jaundice is to exclude the easily diagnosed and fairly common conditions in the first instance, then to await resolution of the jaundice during the next 3 weeks on the assumption that it is physiological, and only if the jaundice persists after that time to pursue further investigations. The threat of kernicterus (see next section) is the important exception to this advice.

Urgent conditions

These include haemolytic diseases, sepsis and metabolic disorders.

Haemolytic disease   Excessive haemolysis of the infant's erythrocytes is usually due to the infant being Rhesus (D) positive, the mother Rhesus negative. If the mother has been sensitized against the D antigen by a previous pregnancy or blood transfusion of Rhesus-positive blood, her anti-D antibodies cross the placenta and attack the infant's erythrocytes. The diagnosis is made by grouping the maternal and infant blood, and by performing the Coombs' test (which detects circulating antibody) on the infant's blood. Very occasionally other blood groups can be responsible and the Coombs test may then be negative.

It is current practice to inject every Rhesus-negative mother with anti-D antibody during the 48 hours after the birth of her baby. If the infant happens to be Rhesus positive and any of its cells reach the maternal circulation, they are destroyed by the injected antibody before they are able to sensitize the mother. This measure has practically eliminated the problem where it has been adequately instituted.

In cases of established haemolytic disease, the mildly affected present with jaundice rather than anaemia. In severe cases, high concentrations of unconjugated bilirubin (above 350 μmol/l, 20 mg/100 ml) can damage the basal ganglia of the brain—*kernicterus*—producing deafness and mental retardation with athetoid movements. To prevent these serious complications it is necessary urgently to perform exchange-transfusion, i.e. alternately to bleed and transfuse the infant in small aliquots until twice the blood volume has been replaced with compatible whole blood.

Sepsis   Sepsis anywhere can interfere with the function of the infantile liver, and any obvious site of infection should be dealt with expeditiously.

Metabolic disorders   *Hypothyroidism* is the most important of the metabolic disorders, partly because it is relatively common (1 in 5000 live births) and partly because the mental retardation it produces can be prevented by early diagnosis.

Cystic fibrosis is also quite common (1 in 2500). Several of the group of diseases due to inborn errors of metabolism (i.e. genetically determined lack of specific enzymes) are associated with neonatal jaundice, although the reason for the jaundice is often not clear. *Galactosaemia* (1 in 40 000) is due to lack of galactose-1-phosphate uridyltransferase, an enzyme essential for the metabolism of galactose, and *hereditary fructose intolerance* (less than 1 in 100 000) is due to the lack of hepatic fructose-1-phosphate aldolase; these conditions should be suspected if routine testing of the infant's urine reveals a reducing substance that is not glucose.

Physiological jaundice
Usually no treatment is necessary while resolution is awaited, i.e. while the concentration of the glucuronyl transferase in the hepatocytes rises to the normal 'mature' level. However, in very premature infants the level of unconjugated bilirubin in the plasma can be reduced either by exposure of the infant to sunlight or artificial blue light (about 450 nm) which acts mainly through photodegradation of bilirubin in the skin, or by making use of the phenomenon of the 'induction' of hepatic enzymes by various agents such as phenobarbitone.

Persistent jaundice
If the jaundice has not resolved in 3 weeks it is unlikely to be physiological, and further investigations should be performed. While there are many causes of neonatal jaundice, some very rare, most can be grouped as *metabolic, hepatitic* or *cholestatic*.
Metabolic To the conditions already mentioned may be added glucose-6-phosphate dehydrogenase deficiency in erythrocytes, which leads to susceptibility to excessive haemolysis in response to various agents such as sulphonamides or salicylates, and thalassaemia and other haemoglobino-pathies. Deficiency of $alpha_1$-antitrypsin—this is a glycoprotein of low molecular weight that is normally synthesized by the liver—causes hepatic damage in a manner that is not clear, but cirrhosis (also sometimes chronic pulmonary disease) develops; however, there is no jaundice since adult haemoglobin is necessary before haemolytic anaemia can develop.
Hepatitis It is uncertain whether viral hepatitis type A occurs in infants, but the type B with its marker antigen is certainly found in infants whose mothers have had the disease in late pregnancy or soon after parturition. Other virus causes include cytomegalovirus, herpes simplex, congenital rubella, Coxsackie B and adenoviruses. Congenital toxoplasmosis is now more common than the very rare congenital syphilitic hepatitis.
Cholestatic As in adults, it can be very difficult to distinguish between intrahepatic and extrahepatic causes. Intrahepatic cholestasis is a feature of neonatal hepatitis or cirrhosis; extrahepatic cholestasis may be due to atresia of the bile ducts or to a choledochal cyst, conditions which are potentially amenable to surgery.
Diagnosis and management of persistent jaundice The history may give an important clue: the mother may have had hepatitis, rubella or herpes of the genital tract; drugs known to be possible causes of jaundice may have been given. In the *examination* little help will be gained unless a site of sepsis is found. Biochemical and haematological investigations diagnose many of the conditions mentioned above, especially the inborn errors of metabolism, while immunological studies are useful for the identification of hepatitis B antigen, syphilis, and rubella and other viruses. The routine liver function tests are, as already mentioned, even less reliable in infants than in adults for differentiating intrahepatic from extrahepatic cholestasis. Even special biochemical tests—such as the fact that phenobarbitone or oral cholestyramine are said to reduce the plasma bilirubin in intrahepatic but not extrahepatic cholestasis, or that less than 10 per cent of a dose of $_{131}$I-labelled Rose Bengal

appears in the stools over 3 days if there is atresia of the bile ducts with complete obstruction—are unreliable. The value of non-invasive newer investigations such as ultrasound, CAT scanning and (in centres where the expertise for investigating such small patients exists) ERCP is presently under evaluation. Finally, resort is made to invasive measures such as hepatic needle biopsy, PTC and laparotomy; these investigations should be done early rather than late because surgery achieves good results only in those who have a laparotomy before 6 weeks. Unfortunately, in most cases of biliary atresia the whole of the extrahepatic and intrahepatic apparatus is involved, even though only in patches, and effective surgery is seldom possible.

A *choledochal cyst* is a spherical enlargement of part or the whole of the common bile duct. Excision where possible is the ideal treatment; otherwise, the cyst is decompressed by anastomosis to the duodenum or jejunum.

Hepatocellular failure

Hepatocellular failure and jaundice are not synonymous terms, even though jaundice is a very common, and clinically the most obvious, feature of hepatocellular failure. As indicated in the previous section, many causes of jaundice are remote from the hepatocyte, and certainly patients with early or mild damage to the liver are not jaundiced.

Three clinical stages are recognized: mild failure; precoma and coma; and acute or fulminant hepatic failure. Two special syndromes that may also arise as a result of damage to the liver—namely, ascites and portal hypertension—are considered in subsequent sections.

Mild hepatocellular failure

There is a general breakdown of health, with *weakness,* ready *fatiguability, anorexia* and *weight loss.* The breath has a sweet, slightly faecal, smell—the *fetor hepaticus.* This presumably indicates a failure of detoxification by the liver of some volatile product of bacterial activity in the gut. A low grade *pyrexia* is sometimes present (there is a failure of the defence mechanisms, and so intercurrent infections including Gram-negative septicaemia may also occur). *Skin changes* are important in diagnosis: *white nails* are due to opacity of the nail beds and are associated with a low plasma albumin; *liver palms* are warm and bright red due to erythema, the colour fading on pressure; and *vascular spiders,* which also blanch on pressure and are confined to the area of drainage of the superior vena cava (i.e. above the nipples) are a red spot (central arteriole) from which radiate several small vessels looking like the legs of a spider.

Spider telangiectases are probably due to an excess of circulating oestrogens, since these hormones are normally destroyed in the liver and 'spiders' are also sometimes found in pregnancy or in patients given oestrogens therapeutically. Other *hormonal effects* associated with oestrogen excess and commonly found in male patients with liver failure include gynaecomastia, testicular atrophy, diminished libido, impotence or even sterility.

Patients tend to have a *hyperkinetic circulation*: the pulse is bounding, the extremities are flushed and warm, cardiac output is raised and there may be an ejection systolic murmur, skin blood flow is increased but renal blood flow is reduced, and in the late stages the blood pressure falls. The reasons for these circulatory changes are not understood. However, arteriovenous shunting is a theoretical possibility, and it is interesting that such shunts have been demonstrated in the pulmonary circulation and seem to be an important factor in the production in the more severe cases of *cyanosis* and associated finger *clubbing*.

Impairment of the liver's powers of protein synthesis is demonstrated by a fall in plasma *albumin* concentration and interference with the blood-clotting mechanism via *prothrombin*. Urea is made in the liver, but its plasma level does not fall until the very late stages—coma and precoma.

Treatment of hepatocellular failure
General   Bed-rest is usually advised, though its value is difficult to prove. Diet is important because anorexia is such a prominent feature: it should be as appetizing as possible, but there are no special requirements except that the alcoholic may benefit from a high intake of protein. Alcohol is not permitted for 1 year after an attack of hepatocellular failure. Anaemia must be treated energetically, if necessary by transfusion. The itching of jaundice is sometimes relieved by cholestyramine, a chemical that binds bile salts.
Specific   These are measures that are aimed at combating the precise cause of the hepatocellular failure. Any drug suspected or known to be causing the liver damage is withdrawn, the commonest being ethyl alcohol. The combination of bed-rest and complete abstinence from alcohol can effect a remarkable improvement in alcoholic hepatitis or even cirrhosis. *Haemochromatosis* is an inborn error of metabolism which results in an excess of iron being absorbed from the diet despite an increasing accumulation of the metal in the tissues. In advanced cases the body contains about 50 g instead of the normal 4 g, and most of the excess is stored in the liver as the pigments ferritin and haemosiderin. The rest is laid down in other organs, including the pancreas, skin and adrenals. Clinical features include tiredness, hepatomegaly, diminished sexual activity, diabetes and skin pigmentation ('bronzed diabetes'). Treatment is by repeated venesection, each 0.5 litre of blood removing about 250 mg iron. Other inborn errors such as *galactosaemia* have been referred to (p. 90); they may respond favourably to withdrawal of the substance that tends to accumulate in the tissues. The liver damage encountered in children in poor (and particularly tropical) countries due to lack of protein (*kwashiorkor syndrome*) responds to treatment with skimmed milk or mixtures of pure amino acids. *Wilson's disease* or *hepatolenticular degeneration* is a rare disease of children and young adults, characterized by cirrhosis, degeneration of the basal ganglia of the brain and greenish-brown rings at the periphery of the cornea—Kayser–Fleischer rings. It is associated with an accumulation of copper in the tissues, and presents either with evidence of liver damage or with neuropsychiatric disturbances such as tremor, grimacing, slurred speech and changes in personality. Treatment is with oral penicillamine, a substance that chelates copper in a soluble form and increases the urinary excretion to more than 1 mg daily (the normal output is less than 80 μg daily).

It must be emphasized that in the majority of patients the aetiology is either unknown or else some factor such as previous viral hepatitis for which no specific treatment is possible.

Precoma and coma

Any type of liver damage, acute or chronic, can produce a neuropsychiatric disturbance that may culminate in coma or death.

Clinical features

The sleep rhythm may be disturbed to the point of inversion, and the patient is apathetic and slow to react to his surroundings. There are changes in personality and a deterioration in intellect. Speech becomes slow and slurred, and familiar objects may not be recognized. Writing deteriorates markedly, especially the ability to keep to a straight line. If the patient is asked to dorsiflex his wrist with the forearm fixed, a flapping tremor is likely to develop at the wrists. Tendon reflexes are usually increased, but disappear in deep coma. Characteristically, the severity of the symptoms fluctuates considerably. At least in the early stages, the effects are completely reversible.

Aetiology

On post-mortem examination of the brain, an increase in the size and number of astrocytes is found in all areas; this very widespread involvement suggests a metabolic cause for the disturbance. Patients with a surgical anastomosis between portal and caval systems (p. 128) are particularly prone to encephalopathy. This suggests that the condition is due to some toxin from the intestine reaching the brain by bypassing the liver, instead of being detoxicated in the liver. Indeed, all patients with hepatic encephalopathy have an abnormal pathway between portal and systemic circulations, whether within the liver itself due to the inability of the cells to perform their normal functions, or to an extrahepatic block such as thrombosis of the portal vein.

Despite much research, the identity of the toxin has not been established, but the fact that high protein diet aggravates and sterilization of the gut alleviates the symptoms suggests that it may be a product of nitrogen metabolism, perhaps the ammonium ions elaborated by micro-organisms within the large bowel.

Treatment

Treatment follows logically from the aetiology. All protein is excluded from the diet as an acute measure, and chronic limitation of protein intake will probably be necessary in the long term. An attack on the gut flora can be instituted by non-absorbable antibiotics such as neomycin, and this is excellent acute-phase treatment; a useful measure for long-term reduction in the absorption of ammonia from the colon is to give oral lactulose in a sufficient thrice-daily dose to produce two semi-solid stools daily. It probably acts by making the stools more acid, thus reducing the formation of absorabable ammonia from the non-absorbable ammonium ion. In severe and unresponsive cases, it may be necessary to resort to surgical procedures such as exclusion and short-circuiting of most of the large bowel by dividing the ileum near its termination, closing the distal end, and anastomosing the proximal end to the sigmoid. In extreme cases liver transplantation can be considered (p. 102).

Acute or fulminant hepatic failure

When the liver fails early in the course of an acute disease, the mortality rate in some series is as high as 80–90 per cent; nevertheless, the potential rewards of efficient treatment are high because such acute changes in the liver are likely to be reversible if only the patient can be kept alive until the noxious influence has worn off.

While almost any agent that attacks the liver can produce this syndrome, the commonest causes are acute viral hepatitis, especially type B; reactions to drugs and chemicals such as halothane, isoniazid, carbon tetrachloride, paracetamol and a component of toadstools; and severe shock, especially in association with septicaemia.

Treatment

The usual management of an unconscious patient is instituted: conscious level is charted and the airway kept clear. So-called 'stress ulceration' of the stomach or duodenum (shallow erosions which can, however; penetrate more deeply and produce severe haemorrhage) is a feature and the stomach should be kept alkaline by passing a nasogastric tube and instilling an antacid such as magnesium trisilicate at hourly intervals, or else by the use of intravenous cimetidine to reduce gastric acid secretion.

Fluid and electrolyte balance is maintained intravenously, and peripheral circulatory failure due to hypovolaemia or (more often) vasodilatation corrected by appropriate infusions. Since the glycogenolysis of glycogen stores within the liver may fail, there is a tendency to hypoglycaemia which must be frequently monitored and corrected by infusion of glucose. Renal failure (the hepatorenal syndrome) due to reduced perfusion of the renal cortex may demand peritoneal or haemodialysis.

Respiratory depression in the later stages requires controlled mechanical ventilation via an endotracheal tube.

A frequent cause of death is the bleeding tendency, and a low prothrombin index is a bad prognostic sign; patients with a value of this index less than 10 per cent of normal rarely survive. The bleeding tendency is treated with intravenous vitamin K_1, fresh blood, fresh-frozen plasma or platelet preparations, according to any detailed deficiencies revealed bv tests.

Finally, there is a group of measures under the general heading of *temporary hepatic support*, designed to perform for the patient those functions that his liver cannot do. They range from exchange blood transfusion or cross-circulation with a healthy donor to the use of charcoal or a porcine, or even a human cadaveric, liver in an extracorporeal circulation. The techniques are not routinely available, and except in a few special centres the results have been of dubious value.

Ascites

Ascites is a collection within the peritoneal cavity of liquid containing the crystalloids of plasma in roughly the same concentrations as in plasma, but proteins in a smaller concentration than in the plasma. It is diagnosed by the physical signs of shifting dullness and a fluid thrill. Percussion in the flanks elicits a dull note with the patient lying supine but when he turns on his side, the opposite (uppermost) side becomes resonant because the ascites gravitates away. A 'fluid thrill' is a shock wave felt by the examiner's hand in one flank when the opposite flank is flicked or tapped; in an obese patient, such a shock wave can be propagated by the subcutaneous tissues, so the test must be done with some object (usually a nurse's forearm) firmly placed on the subject's abdominal wall in the midline so as to damp down any superficial vibrations. It can sometimes be difficult to distinguish ascites from other causes of abdominal distension such as fat, flatus, faeces, fetus or a large, very soft ovarian cyst. Ultrasonography is usually accurate in diagnosing ascites. *Paracentesis abdominis*, the passage of a long needle through the anterior abdominal wall into the peritoneal cavity, yields straw-coloured liquid to confirm the diagnosis.

Aetiology

In essence, ascitic fluid is either an exudate or a transudate from the portal capillaries.

Exudates result from an increased permeability of the capillary walls, permitting a protein-rich liquid to pass through the capillary walls. This occurs in generalized peritonitis (although the clinical picture of ascites is completely overshadowed by more dramatic features such as pain, tenderness and guarding), chronic inflammation such as tuberculosis, and neoplasia, particularly with widespread secondary carcinomatous deposits in the peritoneum.

Transudates have a low protein concentration, less than 20 g/l (2 g/100 ml) compared with the 60–70 g/l of plasma. Excessive transudation results from an imbalance between the hydrostatic pressure directed outwards from the capillary and the osmotic pressure of the plasma proteins attracting liquid from the interstitial space back into the capillary. The factors responsible for ascites thus can be grouped as raised portal pressure and a low plasma concentration of albumin (since the smaller albumin molecule has a greater osmotic activity per unit weight than the larger globulin).

Raised portal capillary pressure may be due to an impediment to the venous return to the heart (congestive cardiac failure, constrictive pericarditis), and the tendency to oedema is then noted in the territories of the systemic as well as those of the portal circulation: the ankles swell and crepitations can be heard at the bases of the lungs. When ascites occurs without oedema elsewhere, it means that either the hepatic veins or some part of the portal venous system are blocked, and in particular that there is hepatocellular damage which has resulted in a low plasma albumin.

Obstruction of the hepatic veins

The resultant clinical picture is called the *Budd–Chiari* syndrome. The liver swells rapidly, becomes hard and palpable, and is very painful because of stretching of the hepatic capsule. Ascites develops rapidly. Histology shows dilatation and pooling in the central sinusoidal zone of the hepatic lobule.

The immediate cause of the obstruction is thrombosis in the hepatic veins, and aetiological factors include polycythaemia and increased clotting tendency (e.g. oral contraceptives), trauma and local neoplastic invasion. In *Jamaican veno-occlusive disease* the block is subendothelial oedema followed by collagen deposition: the causative factor may be ingested in the so-called Bush tea, an infusion prepared from the leaves of an indigenous shrub.

Obstruction of the portal venous circulation

The causes of portal hypertension are detailed separately (p. 98). Those originating within the liver are particularly likely to be associated with a low plasma albumin.

Treatment

Diagnostic paracentesis, removing a small volume of the ascites for cytological and bacteriological investigation, is often necessary, but therapeutic paracentesis, removing most of the liquid, is only required to relieve the severe discomfort of a very rapid accumulation such as may develop with acute occlusion of the hepatic veins.

The mainstays of treatment are a diet with a very low content of sodium (less than 10 mmol (10 mEq) daily if possible) and a daily water intake limited to 1 litre, together with the use of natriuretic diuretics (i.e. those that block the renal mechanisms for conserving sodium).

Portal hypertension

Physiology and pathophysiology

The normal pressure in the portal venous system is about 7 mmHg. The rate of portal blood flow is 1 litre per minute, and since the blood is well oxygenated the resting difference in oxygen content between arterial and portal venous blood is about 2 volumes per cent; the portal system is responsible for no less than 70 per cent of the oxygen supply to the liver Considering the direction of flow in the system, it is no surprise that the pressure in the splenic pulp is a little higher (7–13 mmHg) and that in the hepatic veins a little lower (4–6 mmHg).

An obstruction anywhere in the portal circulation produces a rise in pressure proximal to the block; i.e. the intrasplenic pressure is always above normal. In terms of altered physiology, however, there are three possible sites for the block: *extrahepatic, intrahepatic presinusoidal* and *intrahepatic postsinusoidal.*

In both forms of intrahepatic block the pressure in the right and left branches of the portal vein just before they enter the liver substance is of the same order as the intrasplenic pressure; if, however, the main trunk of the portal vein is obstructed, then the pressure in the branches distal to the block is normal. In all cases of obstruction proximal to the sinusoids, whether extra- or intrahepatic, the pressure in the hepatic veins is normal, but in cases of lesions distorting the architecture of the liver cells themselves, in close relation to the sinusoids, the hepatic vein radicles are compressed to some extent as well as the portal system and the pressure in the hepatic veins is also high.

The hypertension in the portal system results in enlargement of the spleen and the opening of venous channels (that presumably normally lie collapsed) connecting the portal with the systemic circulation so that the trapped blood can ultimately find its way via the venae cavae to the heart.

Clinical features

Collateral ciculation
The most important site is around the cardia of the stomach, where veins in the territory of the left gastric artery anastomose with veins of the diaphragm and oesophagus. The dilated channels lie in the submucosa of the lower end of the oesophagus and upper end of the stomach—the so-called oesophageal varices—where they are susceptible to trauma and an important cause of acute haematemesis and melaena.

A rare but oft-described site is at the umbilicus. The paraumbilical veins of the fetus, running between the umbilicus and the left branch of the portal vein along the free edge of the falciform ligament, collapse after birth but do not disappear. In intrahepatic forms of obstruction they open and bring blood to the umbilicus, whence it continues by a series of subcutaneous dilated veins radiating like the spokes of a wheel and fancifully termed the 'caput Medusae'.

Other sites of collaterals are not clinically apparent (though they may be a nuisance to a surgeon during his dissection): between abdominal organs, such as the liver and spleen, and the contiguous abdominal wall, into the left renal vein, and in the anal canal between the superior haemorrhoidal (portal) and the middle and inferior haemorrhoidal (systemic) veins. Incidentally, the fact that piles are no more common in subjects with than in subjects without portal hypertension suggests that the old explanation that a pile is a dilated vein is not correct (p. 139).

Splenomegaly
An enlarged spleen is the most important single physical sign of portal hypertension. The organ is firm, dull to percussion, and moves downwards and medially when the patient inhales deeply; its characteristic notch may be discernible.

The formed elements of the blood, stagnant within the sinusoids of the enlarged spleen, are subject to its destructive influence to a heightened extent and there results a reduction in concentration of all the cells in the blood—*pancytopenia*. This syndrome is known as *hypersplenism*.

Associated features

The cause of the portal hypertension is often disease of the liver, and therefore a palpable liver and signs of failure of hepatic function (p. 92) are common. Portal hypertension, in combination with the hypoalbuminaemia of hepatic failure, is a potent cause of ascites (p. 96).

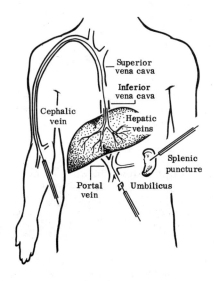

Fig. 6.3 Pressure measurements in the investigation of portal hypertension. A raised pressure in the spleen confirms portal hypertension. If the pressure in the left branch of the portal vein is much less high, the site of the block is extrahepatic; if nearly as high, the site is intrahepatic. In cases of intrahepatic block, if the wedged hepatic vein pressure is almost as high, the block is post sinusoidal; if much lower, the block is presinusoidal.

Investigations (Fig. 6.3)

The pressure in the splenic sinusoids can be measured with a manometer connected to a needle inserted into the spleen by percutaneous puncture. A paraumbilical vein can be found by dissection near the umbilicus, and catheterized to enable the pressure in the left branch of the portal vein to be measured. A catheter passed via a peripheral vein into the inferior vena cava can be manipulated to engage a hepatic vein and progress until it impacts in a hepatic venous tributary: the *wedged hepatic venous pressure* measured via such a catheter is an index of postsinusoidal portal venous pressure. A combination of these measurements allows the site of the obstruction to be categorized. The injection of radio-opaque contrast medium along the needle or catheter at these three sites permits the portal circulation proximal and distal to the block to be visualized (Fig. 6.4). Oesophageal varices are demonstrable by barium swallow (Fig. 6.5) or (better) by oesophagogastroscopy. Where the cause has been demonstrated to be intrahepatic, liver biopsy is likely to be the most useful way of making an exact diagnosis.

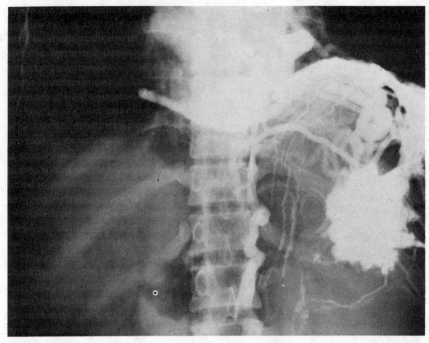

Fig. 6.4 Splenoportal phlebogram. The injected contrast in the splenic pulp is the large lake in the patient's left flank. The splenic vein lies transversely, and is continued across the midline as the commencement of the portal vein. However, there is a complete block in the latter at the line of the tips of the vertebral transverse processes.   (Film kindly provided by Dr John Olney)

Causes

Extrahepatic obstruction

Obliteration of the portal vein may be a congenital anomaly, due to thrombosis within the lumen or to pressure on the wall from without. Thrombosis in the neonatal period may be secondary to portal pyaemia resulting from infection of the umbilicus; this cause is not uncommon in certain cultures where it is customary to dress the umbilical wound at birth with dung. In later life, sepsis may originate at other abdominal (e.g. appendicitis) or even extra-abdominal sites (e.g. osteomyelitis). Thrombosis may also be secondary to blood dyscrasias, such as polycythaemia, or to increased coagulability of the blood due to drugs. Pressure from without may be due to neoplasia of the pancreas or bile ducts, or a large pancreatic pseudocyst (p. 46) resulting from acute pancreatitis.

Intrahepatic presinusoidal obstruction

Viewed world-wide, the commonest cause is probably schistosomiasis (bilharziasis), but viral hepatitis, Hodgkin's disease, primary biliary cirrhosis and poisoning with arsenic are examples of conditions within the liver that obstruct the portal system proximal to the sinusoids.

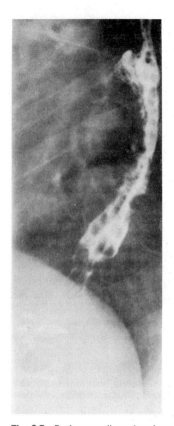

Fig. 6.5 Barium swallow showing oesophageal varices as multiple filling defects.

Intrahepatic postsinusoidal obstruction
In practice the cause is cirrhosis, of any aetiology (p. 89), although an idiopathic form without any obvious cause for the obstruction does rarely occur.

Treatment

Acute haematemesis and melaena
See Chapter 7 for a general discussion of this problem, including the management of bleeding oesophageal varices.

Portal hypertension without acute bleeding
There is no indication for shunt operations in these patients. Conservative measures for liver failure, and if necessary for ascites, are undertaken. Any remediable cause found is treated.

Schistosomiasis
Infestation with the parasite, *Schistosoma*, is very common in many parts of Africa, especially in Egypt and the Sudan and in the countries along the east

coast, in the West Indies and the neighbouring coastal regions of South America, and in some eastern Mediterranean and south-east Asian countries. The male and female forms live in the venous circulation of the colon, and shed ova which are disseminated by the blood stream. Symptoms are produced by the irritant effect of these ova in the tissues.

There are three main varieties: *Schistosoma mansoni* which particularly affects the liver and to a lesser extent the large bowel, *S. Japonicum* which affects small and large bowel, and *S. haematobium* which affects the ureters and bladder.

With all three types, ova are also excreted in the faeces. Further development of the ova into the ciliated larvae or miracidia is facilitated in stagnant water. The miracidia are ingested by snails, the intermediate hosts, in which the miracidia become cercariae, the free-swimming form that is infective for man and can penetrate the intact skin.

Hepatic schistosomiasis

The ova settle in and around the portal venous radicles and excite a steadily progressive periportal fibrosis until eventually the liver is converted into a shrunken and very hard structure. Perhaps because the lesion is predominantly pre- rather than postsinusoidal, hepatocellular function is remarkably well preserved compared with patients in whom the cause of the fibrosis is multinodular cirrhosis. This feature may explain why operations to decompress the portal venous system are associated with a better prognosis in patients with schistosomiasis than in patients with multinodular cirrhosis.

The *diagnosis* of all forms of schistosomiasis depends mainly on the finding of ova in urine or faeces. Rectal mucosal biopsy demonstrates the ova in many patients. Various forms of immunological tests are also available; for example, complement fixation and fluorescent antibody tests.

Treatment is with various antimony preparations (e.g. sodium antimonyl-gluconate for hepatic disease, niridazole for extrahepatic)—particularly in the early stages before the fibrosis has become too dense—and with a variety of surgical operations to deal with mechanical complications of the disease. Under this latter heading fall operations for reducing portal hypertension (p. 128).

Liver transplantation

In a few centres around the world surgeons are working in this field with generally poor, but gradually improving results. The technical problems of the operation, which involves anastomosis of hepatic arteries, portal veins, hepatic veins and bile duct, are formidable but these procedures are nearing standardization. The problems of finding donors, removing the liver from the cadaver before irreversible ischaemic damage has been caused, and preserving the organ during transport and preparation of the patient to receive the graft are still not completely solved. There remains the most important bugbear—rejection of the donor's liver by the recipient's immune processes. Tissue-typing is used to try to ensure the greatest possible measure of compatibility, and the host immune system is suppressed by such agents as corticosteroids and azathioprine.

As yet there are few long-term survivors, so selection of patients for this procedure is necessarily restricted to those known beyond doubt to be suffering from irreversible disease of the liver but otherwise fit. Extensive primary carcinoma of the liver that has not spread elsewhere is one indication.

Further reading

Cotton, P. B. and Williams, C. B. (1980). *Practical Gastrointestinal Endoscopy.* Blackwell Scientific, Oxford.

Hand, B. H. (1976). Presentation and management of stones in the common bile duct. In *Current Surgical Practice*, vol. 1, pp. 114–131. Ed. by G. J. Hadfield and M. Hobsley. Edward Arnold, London.

Marsden, P. D. (Ed.) (1978). *Intestinal Parasites.   Clinics in Gastroenterology 7*, no. 1.

Mowat, A. P. (1979). *Liver Disorders in Childhood.* Butterworths, London and Boston.

Sherlock, S. (1981). *Diseases of the Liver and Biliary System*, 6th edn. Blackwell Scientific, Oxford, London, Edinburgh, Boston, Melbourne.

Sherlock, S. (Ed.) (1980). *Virus Hepatitis.   Clinics in Gastroenterology 9*, no. 1.

Shields, R. (1978). Portal hypertension and bleeding oesophageal varices. In *Current Surgical Practice,* vol. 2, pp. 299–324. Ed. by G. J. Hadfield and M. Hobsley. Edward Arnold, London.

7

Abdominal emergencies related to the alimentary tract

No clinical problem is more potentially taxing than the so-called *acute abdomen*—a patient with abdominal symptoms of acute onset, usually including pain, and possibly produced by a condition threatening life. The general practitioner sees his patient outside the hospital setting, in conditions in which accurate history-taking and physical examination are difficult and special investigations not immediately available, yet he has to decide whether the patient should be sent to hospital or tucked up for the night with reassurance and a placebo.

Acute abdominal symptoms can arise from a generalized disease (e.g. diabetes mellitus, ochronosis or lead colic); or the symptoms and signs may be referred from extra-abdominal organs such as the heart, the lungs or the spine; or again they might originate in intra-abdominal organs outside the alimentary tract (e.g. the kidneys or the abdominal aorta). Nevertheless, the majority of patients are suffering from diseases of the abdominal viscera of the alimentary tract, and this chapter concentrates on these conditions, without specific mention of the important problem of trauma to the abdomen.

There are four main modes of presentation: peritonitis, intestinal obstruction, bleeding from the alimentary tract and massive diarrhoea. Some patients present with a merging of two or more of these major subdivisions, but it is usually easy to assign the patient to one of these four main groups; the last is by far the least common. Peritonitis can be subdivided into generalized, and three localized forms according to whether the symptoms and signs are in the right iliac fossa, the upper abdomen or the left iliac fossa.

Generalized peritonitis

The clinical picture of a patient with established generalized inflammation of the peritoneum is characteristic. The patient complains of severe generalized abdominal pain, much worse on movement, and so he lies still and takes only shallow breaths so that the abdominal wall barely moves with the respiratory excursions. The pain is unremitting, and the only posture that may afford a little relief is flexion of the hips. Abdominal tenderness is also marked, sometimes to the extent that the patient cannot bear the weight of bedclothes or even of his pyjamas, on his anterior abdominal wall. Pallor, sweating and empty superficial veins are usually present, the pulse rate is rapid, the blood pressure may be low and the patient looks anxious. Cyanosis at the periphery, in combination with pallor, may cause a peculiar leaden hue. On gentle palpation it is found that the muscles of the abdomen are in tonic contraction—the usual description is 'board-like rigidity'—and the patient is quite incapable of relaxing these muscles. On auscultation, bowel sounds are absent.

Even though this picture is so characteristic, difficulties do sometimes arise. Soon after the onset, both the abdominal and the generalized signs may be poorly developed and difficult to interpret; chronic steroid and acute opiate administration can mask symptoms, while a few patients are so stoic that the clinician may not appreciate how much pain they are experiencing. Particularly helpful is the sign of generalized *guarding*, elicited best with gentle small movements of flexion at the metacarpophalangeal joints of the examining hand, the interphalangeal joints being kept extended. Small deformities of the anterior abdominal wall are produced, and not much pain, but the reflex tightening of the muscles every time the abdominal wall is deformed is the guarding that is being sought, and generalized guarding (like rigidity) means generalized peritonitis.

In generalized peritonitis the whole of the peritoneum is being severely irritated. The cause, in first instance chemical, is usually the presence of acid or alkaline material containing enzymes in the peritoneal cavity. The usual source is the secretions of the alimentary tract, and the usual route whereby they reach the peritoneal cavity is a breach in the alimentary tract wall—*perforation*. Another, much less common, mechanism is rupture of the wall of the gland producing the alimentary exocrine secretion, such as occurs in acute pancreatitis. Very occasionally the irritant cause is a micro-organism, gaining access to the peritoneum via the blood stream or, in the female, via the genital tract and the Fallopian tubes. The status of *blood* as a cause of acute peritonitis is controversial. It is generally held that blood shed acutely into the peritoneal cavity produces marked irritation. However, most conditions producing intraperitoneal haemorrhage are themselves liable to produce pain and tenderness; for example, the fractured rib that is so often associated with a laceration of the spleen or liver, and the gross distension of the Fallopian tube caused by an ectopic pregnancy. Moreover, there is no doubt that *sometimes* at least, haemoperitoneum is not accompanied by signs of peritoneal irritation, and that the intraperitoneal route can even be used (in infants) for blood transfusion without any obvious discomfort.

Pathophysiological effects

The two principal consequences are *paralytic ileus* and *shock*.

Paralytic ileus
The chemical irritants within the peritoneal cavity interfere with the normal propulsive activity of the bowel (Sanford: *Digestive System Physiology,* Chapter 4)

and peristalsis ceases: this explains the loss of bowel sounds. Swallowed air and secretions of the gastrointestinal tract above the mid-jejunum (the region where net water absorption begins) fail to reach the absorptive area and so abdominal distension arises, producing anorexia and nausea and finally vomiting (compare mechanical intestinal obstruction, p. 115). The loss of electrolytes resulting from vomiting and from distension of the alimentary tract is considered in more detail later (p. 107), but in practice can be considered effectively to be normal saline (i.e. about 150 mmol/l sodium chloride). This loss of saline is one of the elements in the aetiology of the accompanying shock.

Shock

At least in the earlier stages, the principal cause of the reduced tissue perfusion responsible for the rapid thready pulse, hypotension, tachycardia, breathlessness and agitation of the patient with established peritonitis is *hypovolaemia*. One cause of this hypovolaemia is the loss of saline. It is remarkable, however, that shock can be severe even in the absence of marked abdominal distension and vomiting. The reason is that when the peritoneum becomes generally inflamed, its blood vessels dilate and so the capillaries and venules become more permeable: a dilated capillary is a leaky capillary. The consequence is the passage of plasma proteins out of the circulation into the peritoneum itself and also into the interstitial space, accompanied—because of the osmotic effect—by a corresponding volume of water and electrolytes. In other words, there is a loss of plasma from the circulation, just as there is in burns; indeed, at laparotomy on a patient with generalized peritonitis the surgeon finds a considerable effusion within the abdominal cavity, the exact nature of which varies with the cause of the peritonitis but it always contains protein in a concentration of about 40 g/l (4.0 g/100 ml).

Whether the loss is predominantly saline or plasma, or whether it is a mixture of the two, the haemodynamic consequences are due to a fall in the plasma volume and thus in the blood volume. Since there has been no reduction in red cell mass, the *haematocrit* rises. If the loss has been pure plasma, there is no reason for the plasma protein concentration to alter. If, however, the loss has been pure saline, and the plasma volume has shrunk only because it is a part of the whole extracellular space and without any loss of protein from the plasma compartment, then the concentration of the plasma protein rises. Thus serial measurements of the haemocrit and the plasma protein concentration enable calculations of proportionate changes in the plasma volume and the extracellular space respectively.

In many patients there is at least one other cause for shock: a profound generalized capillary vasodilatation resulting from bacterial toxins in bacteraemia or septicaemia, often via the mediation of soluble toxins produced by the micro-organisms. This *toxic* or *septic* shock is a late feature of the average case of chemical peritonitis, but is likely to develop from the outset if a breach in the colon leads to a flood of virulent colonic micro-organisms into the peritoneum. The distinction from hypovolaemic shock can be very difficult, especially as the two types frequently coexist; however, the widespread vasodilatation of septic shock usually produces warm pink extremities rather than the cold pale extremities of hypovolaemia. Fever and rigors may also point towards sepsis.

Management

Management of sequelae
The principle of dealing with *paralytic ileus* is that the bowel is rested. No food is allowed; many authorities recommend that no liquids be permitted, but, taking into account the extreme discomfort produced by drying of the pharynx and oesophagus if this policy is strictly followed, it seems reasonable to allow, say, 30 ml water hourly, an amount that is tiny in proportion to the rate of secretions into the alimentary tract. Nasogastric aspiration is instituted so as to reduce distension, thereby reducing nausea and preventing vomiting. The basic daily requirements of water and electrolytes are given by intravenous infusion. Under no circumstances should parasympathomimetic drugs be given in an effort to stimulate peristalsis: the bowel will start to work again once the peritonitis has been cured and its effects on motility have worn off.

With regard to *shock*, all patients with peritonitis have some degree of hypovolaemic shock; important questions are the relative importance of plasma loss and saline loss, and the possibility that septic shock is also present. Thus all patients require expansion of the plasma volume: logically this expansion should be achieved with normal saline (or a similar solution such as Hartmann's) for losses due to distension and vomiting, and by plasma or plasma-substitutes such as Haemaccel for peritoneal exudation. Pointers to the loss include symptoms and signs such as the severity of nausea and vomiting, loss of skin elasticity as a measure of extracellular depletion, the duration and severity of the peritonitis as judged by the local abdominal signs, and the degree of impairment of renal function as assessed by the blood urea and the urine volume and specific gravity. The more profound the disturbance in renal and haemodynamic terms compared with the evidence of saline losses, the more likely is a substantial loss of plasma: 1 litre of plasma lost out of the normal 3 litres has a much greater effect than 1 litre of saline lost out of the 12–15 litres of the extracellular space. Loss in plasma results in a rise in haematocrit but no change in plasma protein concentration, whereas a reduction in plasma volume because of a contraction of the whole extracellular compartment (of which the plasma is a specialized portion) due to saline loss results in a *rise* in plasma protein concentration.

Some authorities advocate crystalloid rather than colloid solutions for replacing plasma losses. However, to expand the plasma volume by 1 litre with Hartmann's solution requires about 4 or 5 litres, so the plasma is replenished only at the expense of overfilling the extracellular space. This probably does not matter in fit, healthy young subjects, but the increased hydrostatic pressure in the interstitial space can lead to exudation of water and electrolytes into the pulmonary alveoli and this probably is an important factor in causing the pulmonary collapse and consolidation which often occurs in severely shocked patients treated exclusively with crystalloids ('shock lung').

Any suspicion of sepsis should lead to sending of blood samples for immediate bacteriological examination of smears and also for culture, both aerobic and anaerobic. However, the danger of septic shock is so great that if there is clear evidence of systemic disturbance (pyrexia, rigors), antibiotics should be started without waiting for the results of these investigations. The exact choice of antibiotics must depend on information about the current likely organisms. However, at least two, and maybe three, antibiotics should always be used together so as to restrict the emergence of resistant strains, the dosage being high enough to produce effective levels in the tissues. Anaerobic as well as aerobic organisms should be borne in mind; metronidazole for the anaerobes and gentamicin for the aerobes is a popular mixture.

Treatment of the cause
The peritoneum, with a good blood supply, has remarkable powers of recuperation and has little difficulty in recovering from the effects of a chemical, or even a bacteriological invasion provided that the attack is brief. It is a *continuing* insult that is dangerous. Since the route of attack is usually via a breach in the wall of a hollow viscus, the standard treatment of peritonitis must include laparotomy in order both to evacuate the irritant material and to seal the leak. A sucker is used to aspirate the contents of the peritoneum, which is also washed out with normal saline in liberal quantities. The method of sealing the leak depends on the organ affected and the cause. The commonest causes are perforation of a peptic (duodenal or gastric) ulcer, rupture of an acutely inflamed appendix, and rupture of a pericolic inflammatory mass that has developed through a small, localized leak at the site of a diverticulum, usually one of many in the sigmoid region. These three major causes usually produce symptoms and signs that are at first localized to the epigastrium, right iliac and left iliac fossae, respectively, and are therefore considered in more detail later, under the heading of localized peritonitis. First, however, the influence of plain x-rays of the abdomen on diagnosis, and the possibility that the clinical picture is due to acute pancreatitis on the management, are discussed.

Plain abdominal x-rays
The erect and supine plain abdominal x-rays are valuable in the confirmation of the paralytic ileus. The erect film demonstrates gas/liquid levels in the dilated loops of bowel, while the supine film shows more clearly the anatomy of the bowel and indicates that both the small and the large bowel are distended, the latter right down to the anal canal.

Free gas in the peritoneal cavity, usually as a gas/liquid shadow beneath the diaphragm in an erect film, confirms the diagnosis of perforation, but absence of such evidence cannot rule out that diagnosis. Not all patients with a perforated peptic ulcer have this radiological sign, nor does the presence of the sign indicate that the leak is necessarily in an *upper* abdominal viscus.

Acute pancreatitis
This condition can produce clinical features identical to those of generalized peritonitis due to perforation, yet its management should usually be non-operative.

Aetiology The pancreas secretes powerful enzymes which break down fats (*lipases*), proteins (*proteases*) and carbohydrates (*amylases*) and many others including *elastase* that attacks elastic tissue. Within the pancreas they exist as inactive precursors; for example, trypsinogen, the zymogen of the active protease trypsin. If the zymogens are activated within the pancreas itself, instead of only after secretion into the duodenal lumen, autodigestion of the pancreas occurs. Trypsin, once formed from trypsinogen, can release the other enzymes from their precursors. When the walls of acini on the surface of the pancreas are digested, the enzymes flood the peritoneal cavity and a generalized peritonitis results. In the most severe cases there is a particular destruction of blood vessels (elastase) with the formation of a haematoma which provides more substrate for the proteases and adds ischaemia to the other destructive elements; the result is *haemorrhagic necrotizing pancreatitis*, which occurs in only 5 per cent of cases but has an 80 per cent mortality.

In experimental animals, acute pancreatitis can be produced by the injection of mixtures of bile and trypsin into the pancreatic duct at a pressure of 70 cmH$_2$O. Such pressures rupture the walls of the acini, extravasation of this mixture into the interstitial fluid activates complement, phospholipase C is formed as a result, and this agent destroys the plasma membrane of acinar cells and the zymogen granules that contain the inactive precursors—with their release and subsequent activation. The same mechanism is probably involved in *gallstone pancreatitis*. This is the commonest form diagnosed in England (about half the cases); since gallstones can usually be found in the stools of someone who has just had acute pancreatitis and since the patient usually has a common channel at the termination of his common bile and pancreatic ducts, it is likely that the attack is initiated by a gallstone impacted temporarily in the common channel of bile and pancreatic ducts, thereby obstructing the outlet of the pancreatic duct. The patient takes a meal, the pancreas is stimulated to secrete alkali and enzymes, the gall bladder to contract, and the stage is set for the forceful reflux of bile at high pressure into the actively secreting pancreas.

The other major cause of acute pancreatitis is alcohol. In France and the United States, alcohol is a more common cause of acute pancreatitis than gallstones. The mechanism is unknown.

Acute pancreatitis may result from obstruction of the pancreatic duct by a carcinoma or by mechanical disturbance resulting from operations on the stomach or duodenum. Other associated conditions include renal failure, hypercalcaemia and hyperlipoproteinaemia types I and V.

Clinical features The pain usually starts in the epigastrium, although it eventually spreads over the whole abdomen in the more severe cases. In *onset*, it is more gradual than the usual catastrophic suddenness of the perforation of a peptic ulcer. Other features which should alert the clinician to the possibility of this condition include a history of gallstones or of alcoholism, a raised serum amylase concentration during the first 24 hours and a subsequent rise in urinary amylase sometime during the second and third days, and a depressed calcium concentration in the plasma. The serum amylase concentration is normal in 5 per cent of patients with the condition, and very high values normally considered to be diagnostic may occur with other conditions (including perforated peptic ulcer!) in 5 per cent. However, in patients with acute pancreatitis there is a failure of renal tubular reabsorption of plasma amylase, and attempts have recently been made to improve the diagnostic accuracy by comparing its clearance to that of creatinine. The ratio of the amylase to the creatinine clearance is obtained by measuring amylase and creatinine concentrations in simultaneous serum and urine samples and calculating:

$$\frac{\text{urine amylase}}{\text{serum amylase}} \times \frac{\text{serum creatinine}}{\text{urine creatinine}} \times 100$$

The normal value is 3 per cent, while it is about twice this in patients with acute pancreatitis. Ultrasonography may demonstrate gallstones or a swollen pancreas.

The release of enzymes produces not only peritoneal exudation of protein-rich liquid with a rise in haematocrit (but no change in plasma chloride concentration), but also fat necrosis (this contributes to hypocalcaemia, although there is also an unexplained disturbance of parathyroid function), discoloration in the flank (Grey Turner's sign) and umbilical region (Cullen's sign) due to tracking of haematoma along the retroperitoneal plane. A pleural effusion containing a high amylase concentration is common.

Treatment   There is no specific pharmacological treatment. The enzyme-inhibitor aprotinin (Trasylol) and glucagon have both been tried but there is no evidence that they work. Two-thirds of cases are only of mild or moderate severity, and supportive treatment—nasogastric suction for the ileus and infusions of plasma and saline for the oligaemia plus pethidine for pain—are adequate. After recovery, a search is made for gallstones and these are treated by the appropriate operation, while heavy drinkers are advised to abstain. The problem lies with the severe (haemorrhagic) cases. Some authorities advocate a diagnostic peritoneal tap which confirms the presence of enzymes in the liquid and also demonstrates whether it is bloody. There is some evidence that the one-third of patients in the severe category do better if the needle employed for the tap is then used to perform peritoneal dialysis to wash out the enzymes. For haemorrhagic necrotizing pancreatitis only, a few centres are exploring the value of a surgical operation during the acute stage, to remove the sloughing tail and body of the pancreas. This is heroic surgery, and the results are difficult to evaluate.

Localized peritonitis

Right iliac fossa

Localized pain, tenderness and guarding in the right iliac fossa are tantamount to a working diagnosis of acute appendicitis, and should lead to immediate exploration of the right lower quadrant of the abdomen via a gridiron incision.

This dogmatic statement is made to emphasize that acute appendicitis is by far the most common condition producing this clinical picture, and that the penalties for the patient of a surgeon not operating an acute appendicitis are overwhelmingly greater than those for operating and finding some other condition, or even no abnormality.

Clinical features said to support a diagnosis of acute appendicitis include a history of a recent disturbance of bowel habit, anorexia, nausea or vomiting, pain starting centrally and colicky in nature but moving to the right iliac fossa and becoming continuous, and various physical signs such as fetor oris, a furred tongue and crossed iliac fossa tenderness (pain in the right iliac fossa produced by pressure on the left). However, many patients with acute appendicitis have none of these features.

In the same way, many features said to militate against the diagnosis, such as hunger, pyrexia greater than 39°C (102°F), white cells in the urine, can all be present.

The treatment is appendicetomy, and the surgeon's aim should be to perform this operation before the appendix has perforated and given rise to generalized peritonitis with its risk of complications such as abscesses in the wound or the pelvis or under the diaphragm, septicaemia and portal pyaemia. Remember that many patients still die from acute appendicitis, and that, in female patients, a very important and distressing late sequel of peritonitis is infertility.

The *pathogenesis* in about 90 per cent of cases is obstruction of the lumen of the appendix, usually by a faecolith, and often at a site where the appendix is kinked by a congenital peritoneal adhesion. The underlying *aetiology* is unknown, but is related to life in so-called modern Western civilization. The condition became prominent in Western Europe and America just before 1900; it remains rare in developing countries while their inhabitants adhere to traditional customs and eating habits, but it becomes more common when the Western style of living is introduced. Intriguingly, there appears to be a recent reduction in incidence in the United Kingdom, but the reasons are unknown.

Epigastrium

There are two common causes of peritoneal irritation confined to the epigastrium: *acute cholecystitis* and *perforated peptic ulcer*. For acute pancreatitis, see p. 108.

The management of both cholecystitis and perforation can be either conservative or operative. Most clinicians would agree that operative treatment is preferable for perforation, but there is controversy about cholecystitis: in North America the accepted management is early (not necessarily immediate; perhaps on the next available list) operation, whereas in the United Kingdom the usual policy is conservatism in the first instance. However, there is an increasing trend in Britain towards early operation.

In the majority of patients it is not difficult to distinguish between these two conditions. A history of a proven peptic ulcer or of suggestive symptoms, a very sudden rather than more gradual onset, an early spread of the signs of peritoneal irritation (with a continuance of a leak into the lesser sac, the irritant fluid escapes into the greater sac), often associated with absence of bowel sounds, all strongly suggest perforation. Gas under the diaphragm of course confirms that a hollow viscus has perforated. On the other hand, a history of gallstones, pain and tenderness in the right upper quadrant rather midline, tenderness on pressure under the right costal margin increased by deep inspiration (the characteristic catch in the breath at the extreme of inspiration is *Murphy's sign*), a palpable mass in the region of the gall bladder, the absence of true guarding, the presence of bowel sounds, and clinical or biochemical evidence of jaundice all point towards the gall bladder as the seat of the trouble. Ultrasound is particularly useful since it is reliable for the demonstration of stones in, or distension of, the gall bladder.

Conservative management
The principles are: (1) empty the stomach and keep it empty by nasogastric aspiration—this relieves vomiting due to paralytic ileus, reduces duodenal acidification and thereby the stimulation of the gall bladder to contract, and (in cases of perforation) minimizes further soiling of the peritoneal cavity; (2) restore and maintain water and electrolyte balance by suitable infusions; (3) control pain, if necessary by opiates; (4) use antibiotics if there is evidence of septic absorption (pyrexia, rigors); (5) continue with conservative management only so long as there is no suggestion of deterioration—evidence of deterioration includes a rising pulse rate and falling blood pressure despite apparently adequate transfusion, increasing pyrexia, pain or tenderness, spread of the signs of peritoneal irritation and disappearance of bowel sounds if they had been present. With this regimen, the majority of patients with acute cholecystitis will settle, and many patients with a perforation will also doubtless respond although this policy is not recommended as a routine. After recovery from this acute episode the patient is fully investigated, the definitive diagnosis made and treatment advised along lines indicated elsewhere (p. 31 for gallstones; p. 56 for peptic ulcer).

Operative management
Emergency operations for perforated peptic ulcer must seal the leak to prevent further contamination of the peritoneum, and clean out any foreign material from the peritoneal cavity. In selected cases the surgeon may consider performing an operation to cure the peptic ulcer diathesis at the same time.

Sealing the leak is usually readily achieved in a case of perforated duodenal ulcer by stitching an omental patch over the perforation. There can be more difficulty with a perforated gastric ulcer, and in any case a biopsy should be performed in case the lesion is a carcinoma. If the patient has a long previous history of peptic ulcer or the callous appearance of the surroundings of the ulcer suggest chronicity, and if the patient's general condition is satisfactory and the surgeon is experienced in gastric operations, it is reasonable to proceed immediately with a vagotomy or partial gastrectomy.

Early laparotomy for acute cholecystitis is meant to achieve cholecystectomy, peroperative cholangiography and, if indicated, exploration of the common bile duct, exactly as in routine operations for gallstones (p. 32). The fear that the dissection of the cystic duct and artery and the common bile and hepatic ducts in the region of the neck of the gall bladder would be made difficult and dangerous by inflammatory adhesions and oedema has inhibited British surgeons from undertaking this operation in the acute stage. However, the danger seems to be less than imagined, and the technique in most cases well within the capacity of an experienced surgeon. If extreme difficulty is experienced, the bladder is decompressed by drainage to the exterior (cholecystostomy), preferably with digital dislodgement of the stone in Hartmann's pouch that has caused the acute cholecystitis, if this manoeuvre proves possible. Six weeks later, when the local inflammation has subsided, elective cholecystectomy is performed.

In those being treated conservatively for acute cholecystitis, if operation becomes necessary because of deterioration of the patient's condition, it is performed. Cholecystostomy is usually required, but even in these cases cholecystectomy is sometimes safe.

Left iliac fossa

In patients with tenderness and guarding in the left lower quadrant of the abdomen, the source of the leak is nearly always the sigmoid colon, the pathology nearly always *diverticular disease* or *carcinoma*, with the former more common.

Diverticular disease describes anatomical deformity and also a related functional disturbance with complications arising therefrom. The anatomical deformity is multiple diverticula of the mucous membrane through the muscle coat of the large bowel, apparently through points of weakness where the blood vessels penetrate the muscular wall. The diverticula are concentrated in the sigmoid colon and the highest part of the rectum, but they sometimes extend proximally and even, rarely, reach the caecum. There appears to be no relationship between this condition and either *solitary* diverticula of the colon or any other part of the intestine, or the multiple diverticulosis that can affect the jejunum. The functional disturbance, also maximal in the sigmoid, is overactivity of the colonic musculature, evidenced by a considerable work-hypertrophy of the taeniae, and resulting in an increased intraluminal pressure.

Whether the functional disturbance produces the anatomical abnormality (as would appear reasonable) is not known; but the abnormality is common: one-third of patients over the age of 50 undergoing a barium enema examination have some degree of colonic diverticulosis.

The relationship between diverticula and *chronic* symptoms is unclear. Constipation is accepted either as the cause of the high pressure or as the result of excessive drying of the faeces in stagnant, high pressure compartments of the colon. With regard to acute symptoms we are on firmer ground. Infection becomes established in the stagnant faecal contents of a diverticulum, and erodes either a neighbouring artery to produce a severe rectal haemorrhage (a rare but very dramatic event) or the wall of the diverticulum itself. In the latter case, should the perforation occur freely into the general peritoneal cavity the result is general peritonitis of sudden onset. More often, however, the inflammatory process has been low grade and chronic so that there has been time for adhesions to be formed to neighbouring structures such as the great omentum, coils of small bowel, bladder or uterus. Thus when the leak occurs it produces a variably walled off pericolic abscess rather than general peritonitis, and signs of localized peritoneal irritation with or without a palpable mass.

Carcinoma of the colon is considered more fully elsewhere (p. 142), but it, too, can produce either free perforation or a localized pericolic abscess.

Management

Since most cases of left iliac fossa peritonitis are due to diverticular disease and most cases of rupture of the colon due to diverticular disease produce in the first instance a localized pericolic abscess, it is logical to start treatment along conservative lines. If the patient fails to improve, or deteriorates, laparotomy is necessary, and appropriate antibiotics should be started before the operation.

At laparotomy it can be difficult or impossible to decide whether the basic lesion is diverticulitis or carcinoma. The first principle of the emergency management is to prevent any continuing leak into the peritoneal cavity. If possible without undue danger to neighbouring structures such as the ureter, the affected sigmoid loop is mobilized and resected (Fig. 8.3). Sometimes it is safe to perform an immediate end-to-end anastomosis to restore continuity, at the same time diverting the faecal stream from the region of the anastomosis by making a transverse colostomy. Often the peritonitis is so severe that it seems likely the anastomosis will fail to heal, and then the proximal cut end of colon is brought out as a temporary colostomy in the left iliac fossa and the distal cut end is brought out beside it as a double-barrelled colostomy (Paul–Mikulicz operation) or closed and left in the pelvis (Hartmann's operation). If mobilization of the colon seems unwise, there is no alternative to a diverting transverse colostomy and leaving a drain to the site of the leak.

Hartmann's procedure is followed several weeks later, when all the inflammation has subsided, by a second operation to anastomose the descending colon to the stump of rectum, while transverse colostomy is followed similarly by a definitive sigmoid colectomy (second stage) and a month later by closure of the transverse colostomy (third stage). Once the sigmoid, where the main bulk of the diverticula are concentrated, has been resected, it is uncommon to get any further trouble from any diverticula present more proximally in the colon.

If the peritonitis settles on conservative management, there remains the problem of preventing further attacks. The decision to advise a definitive operation will clearly depend on several features such as age and physical fitness, but in general one attack of severe left iliac fossa pain and tenderness is a reasonable indication. The standard operation is sigmoid colectomy when the inflammation has subsided, with immediate end-to-end anastomosis, protected possibly by a transverse colostomy.

Intestinal obstruction

Complete obstruction to the alimentary tract is incompatible with life. Obstruction in the oesophagus is considered in Chapter 2, and this section concerns the rest of the gastrointestinal tract. Apart from the very rare condition of *hourglass stenosis* in the mid-portion of the stomach, due to cicatrization induced by a benign gastric ulcer, the first point below the oesophagus at which obstruction commonly arises is in the region of the pylorus. From that point to the anus itself, obstruction can occur at any point along the alimentary tract.

Genesis of clinical features

The *symptoms* consist of some combination of anorexia, nausea and vomiting on the one hand, with abdominal distension and constipation on the other. In addition, most patients with intestinal obstruction complain of abdominal pain which is characteristically colicky (i.e. intermittent) in nature.

The main *physical signs* are distension, some disturbance of the bowel sounds on auscultation (they are either absent or increased), and evidence of some disturbance of body water and electrolytes. Specific signs associated with the particular cause of the obstruction will be considered later.

The crucial *investigation* is a set of plain x-rays of the abdomen with the patient both erect and supine. Measurements to assess any deficiency of the body fluids and electrolytes are also very important.

The details of this clinical picture and the rationale of management become much simpler when considered in the light of disturbances of physiology.

Symptoms

In health, the aqueous contents of the alimentary tract at any point represent a dynamic equilibrium between secretion into the lumen and absorption from the lumen (Sanford: *Digestive System Physiology*, Chapter 5). Secretion exceeds absorption in the upper tract down to about the mid-small bowel; beyond that point absorption outweighs secretion. The net secretion into the upper portion is large: 24-hour quantities have been assessed at about 750 ml for saliva, 1500 ml for gastric juice, 1 litre for pancreatic juice, and so on. The total net secretion is probably about 10 litres in 24 hours. Since the output of water in the faeces is normally less than 0.5 litre, the rest of this volume must be absorbed. Probably only about 2 litres reach the large bowel, and so it is evident that the distal small bowel has the very important task of reabsorbing more than 6 litres of water.

The maximal disturbance of the body fluids is likely to be produced by obstruction at the point where net secretion changes to net absorption; i.e. somewhere along the proximal third of the jejunum. The whole of the net secretion above that point is still entering the bowel but is not reaching those areas where it should be absorbed. The accumulated secretion stays in the loops of bowel above the obstruction and produces abdominal distension and a feeling of satiety which progresses to nausea and vomiting.

The higher the obstruction, the earlier and more prominent the vomiting (because there is less bowel available to accommodate the collected liquid), while abdominal distension becomes less prominent. Since the large bowel is unaffected and contains its normal large load of faeces, there is probably little disturbance of bowel habit; certainly the patient will not have had time to notice constipation during the very few hours before he is seriously ill with depletion of the body fluids.

By contrast, obstruction low in the large bowel is likely to be associated with constipation once the short segment of colon below the obstruction has been emptied of faeces. The really significant feature is that the patient passes no flatus. Absence of the passage of flatus is called *absolute constipation*, a rather misleading term because it seems to imply that no faeces must be passed, but this is not intended. Nausea and vomiting in large bowel obstruction are likely to be much less prominent than in small bowel obstruction because considerable reabsorption of liquid has taken place from the ileum and the colon proximal to the obstruction. Distension remains a prominent feature, but due to swallowed air and microbial gas rather than trapped secretion.

The distended bowel above the obstruction is stimulated to increased peristaltic activity and this is associated with intermittent cramping pain. This pain is vaguely localized, placed symmetrically about the midline; in high small bowel obstruction it tends to be epigastric while in large bowel obstruction it tends to be hypogastric. Each attack may be associated with a gradual increase and a gradual diminution, but the most important feature is that there is complete remission, with freedom from pain, between the attacks. True colicky pain is unusual in large bowel obstruction, where the main pain is often felt in the right iliac fossa and is probably due to distension of the caecum—thin-walled in its musculature compared with the rest of the colon—because the ileocaecal valve may be competent and prevent decompression by reflux into the small bowel.

Paralytic ileus, due to an absence of normal peristaltic activity, modifies the picture, particularly by the elimination of colicky abdominal pain. However, the condition producing the ileus may itself be associated with pain; for example, the generalized constant pain of peritonitis (p. 104).

For the genesis of the signs of disturbance of body fluids, see p. 106 and below.

Signs

Abdominal *distension* is a sign as well as a symptom. In cases of low large bowel obstruction, *percussion* of the distended abdominal wall yields a *tympanitic* note. On *auscultation*, the abdomen is silent in cases of paralytic ileus, but in cases of mechanical obstruction the increased peristalsis results in frequent bowel sounds characterized by repetitive runs and marked gurgling or tinkling noises due to the vigorous churning of the contained liquid with swallowed air. These are 'obstructive bowel sounds'.

The signs of *depletion of the body fluids* in simple intestinal obstruction (as distinct from strangulation-obstruction) are related to depletion of the extracellular compartment because the losses from the alimentary tract are effectively normal saline. Thus there is a particular loss of skin elasticity and, in severe cases, depressed tone in the eyeballs. The other disturbance are those of oligaemic shock.

Investigations

The gastrointestinal tract contains not only liquid but also swallowed gas, to which is added a small quantity by fermentation due to gastrointestinal micro-

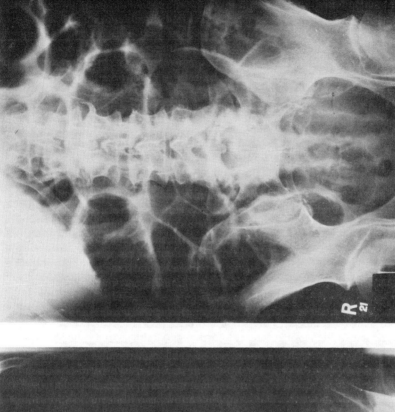

(a)

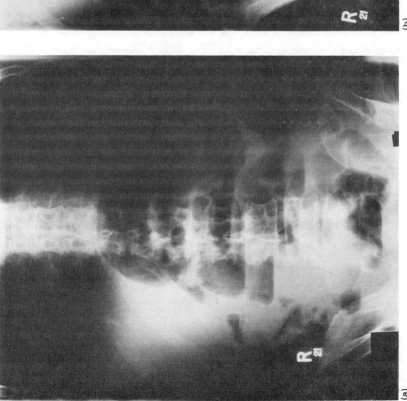

(b)

Fig. 7.1 Small bowel obstruction: plain abdominal x-rays. (a) Erect. The multitude of fairly short gas/liquid horizontal levels and the disposition of the dilated loops of bowel in the central abdomen rather than in the periphery are characteristic of small bowel obstruction. (b) Supine. This view is better for showing details of the anatomy of the dilated loops than is the erect. The lines (valvulae conniventes) transversely crossing the bowel shadows cross the whole lumen and do not greatly indent the edges where they meet the latter. These characteristics are typical of small rather than large bowel. Where the lines are close together (in the right upper quadrant) the bowel is jejunum; where further apart (in the right lower quadrant), ileum.

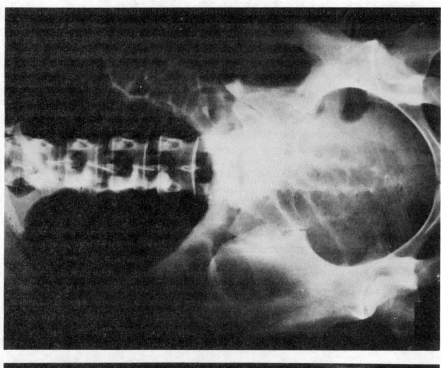

(a)

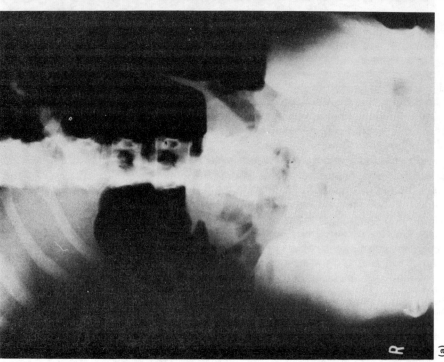

(b)

Fig. 7.2 Large bowel obstruction: plain abdominal x-rays. (a) Erect. The disposition of the horizontal gas/liquid levels around the periphery of the abdomen—the flanks and the epigastrium—suggests large rather than small bowel obstruction. (b) Supine. The dilated ascending, transverse and descending colon can be clearly seen. The horizontal cross-markings (haustrations) do not extend across the whole width of the lumen, but they are associated with indentation of the outline of the bowel (particularly well seen near the lower border of the most dependent part of the transverse colon). These features are typical of large bowel obstruction.

organisms. In the normal subject, the amount of liquid in the small bowel far outweighs the volume of gas and so one does not normally see gas in the small bowel. On the other hand, most of the liquid has been absorbed by the time the large bowel is reached and there is increased production of gas from micro-organisms; for these reasons, it is normal to see gas throughout the large bowel.

In small bowel obstruction, the significant radiological features are dilated loops of small bowel containing multiple air/liquid levels and an absence of gas in the large bowel (Fig. 7.1). In large bowel obstruction, the typical feature is gaseous distension of the large bowel with some fluid levels, but the distension cannot be traced downwards into the rectum as the normal gas shadows should be, and in some cases the demarcation at the lower limit of the gas is quite accurate in showing the point of obstruction (Fig. 7.2). Should the ileocaecal value be competent, there may be little or no abnormality to be seen in the small bowel, but in many patients with large bowel obstruction this valve is incompetent and one then sees loops of distended small bowel with air/gas fluid levels just as in small bowel obstruction.

The supine film is best to demonstrate whether the loops seen are small bowel or large, while the erect film demonstrates the air/liquid levels. Loops of small bowel tend to be centrally placed with the valvulae conniventes visible as straight lines traversing the whole width of the bowel, while large bowel tends to be peripherally placed and shows the indentations called haustrations that do not usually run across the whole width of the bowel.

Management

The clinician has to answer five questions in every case of possible intestinal obstruction. First, is the patient obstructed? There should be no doubt after the plain x-rays have been taken. Secondly, is the obstruction mechanical or paralytic? Colicky pain and increased bowel sounds should leave one in no doubt. Thirdly, is the obstruction in the small bowel or the large bowel, because this differentiation has an important effect on management. The clinical picture in combination with the radiological examination should make this question easy to answer.

The fourth question is crucial: is the obstruction *simple* in nature or is there an associated element of *strangulation*? Strangulation implies circumferential pressure at the neck of the portion of tissue, such that the venous return is preferentially obstructed so that the part becomes engorged with stagnant blood. If unrelieved, a process of wet gangrene ensues, and if the part includes bowel then perforation and general peritonitis become inevitable. A diagnosis of strangulation is thus tantamount to a call for an immediate operation to relieve the obstruction and the strangulation.

Strangulation must be suspected if, either instead of or in addition to colicky abdominal pain, the patient complains of a continuous background of abdominal pain. Other features such as pyrexia, polymorphonuclear leucocytosis, or signs of local peritonitis such as guarding may also be present but their absence does not counterweigh the presence of continuous pain.

The fifth question is, does the patient show the signs of a disturbance of water and electrolytes? In simple intestinal obstruction, the losses are in effect pure saline, but in strangulation-obstruction, the distended capillaries leak large quantities of protein-rich liquid into the tissues and an element of plasma loss is added. In consequence, the patient has more severe signs and symptoms of shock and a haematocrit increased more than one might have expected.

The principles of management may be summarized under six headings, as follows.

1. *Nasogastric suction*
Efficient nasogastric aspiration prevents vomiting, relieves nausea, and reduces abdominal distension and discomfort. Measurement of the volume of aspirate gives information about the magnitude of losses from the alimentary tract.

2. *Replenish any depletion*
Simple intestinal obstruction depletes the extracellular fluid because the secretions of the gastrointestinal tract are effectively physiological (i.e. 9 g/l, isotonic or 'normal') saline. Losses from the stomach are acidic while losses from the intestine are alkaline. Nevertheless, any consequent disturbance of acid–base balance can be corrected by the kidneys secreting urine of the opposite reaction. The important thing is to restore and maintain renal function by restoring the circulating volume so that these adjustments can be made by the kidney. To estimate the volume of saline required to reconstitute the extracellular space, the clinician assumes that a very seriously depleted patient with sunken eyeballs, lax skin and anuria requires 6 litres of physiological saline while a patient with just detectable depletion requires 2 litres; anyone between these two clinical extremes requires 4 litres.

Patients with strangulation require colloid (i.e. plasma or a plasma substitute) in a volume of about 1 litre in addition to any saline requirements they might have.

These procedures to restore the balance of water and electrolytes must be started, and in patients with severe depletion at least half-completed, before there is any question of anaesthesia for a surgical operation.

3. *Indications for* **urgent** *operation*
The chief indication for operation is a clinical suspicion of strangulation. In cases of large bowel obstruction, the finding of marked tenderness and guarding in the right iliac fossa suggests that rupture of the caecum may be imminent and occasionally this feature demands early operation.

4. *The general rule is to* **operate**
This principle is all-important. Its importance is sometimes obscured by the fact that operation should be delayed for resuscitation and also for reasons given in the next paragraph, but the idea that intestinal obstruction can be expected to be cured without a surgical operation is dangerous.

5. *Prerequisites for operation*
It is again emphasized that resuscitation must be adequate. Patients with simple small bowel obstruction thought to be due to postoperative adhesions

(below) are treated by nasogastric aspiration and intravenous fluids without opiates, and reassessed with regard to the completeness of the obstruction each 24 hours by clinical examination and plain x-rays of the abdomen. Provided that the assessment shows a definite improvement, conservative management may be continued. Any hint of strangulation or any failure to improve in any 24-hour period must be treated by operation. In patients with large bowel obstruction, one and maybe two enemas are given before taking the patient to theatre. There are two reasons for this. First, in a patient with a constricting lesion of the left side of the colon the final obstructive agent may be a mass of solid faeces at the construction ring and this may be dislodged by the enema; the obstruction is thus relieved and time is given for proper preoperative investigations of the cause of the obstruction before laparotomy. Secondly, there is a condition of *pseudo-obstruction of the colon* which closely mimics organic left-sided obstruction but for which no organic cause can be found at laparotomy. Such cases usually deflate after enemas and washouts and operation is avoided.

6. *What to do at operation*
A removable obstruction is removed, and an irremovable obstruction must be bypassed in some way. If these manoeuvres result in a loss of continuity of the gastrointestinal tract, then continuity can be immediately restored by direct anastomosis if one arm at least of the anastomosis is small bowel. However, if the two cut ends of bowel are both large bowel, it is dangerous to attempt an immediate anastomosis in the presence of the pathophysiological changes in the bowel produced by obstruction. Some form of colostomy is therefore necessary whereby the proximal limb is brought out to the skin surface of the abdominal wall, and the distal limb is similarly dealt with or is closed and left within the abdominal cavity if it will not reach the skin.

Causes

The immediate cause of intestinal obstruction often cannot be diagnosed and treatment must be instituted in terms of the general principles given above. The following paragraphs highlight a few of the more common and interesting conditions.

Strangulated external hernia
The clinical features of a strangulated external hernia are a tense tender lump lacking a cough impulse, and situated at an external hernial orifice. The diagnosis should be obvious, but it is easy to miss a small lump in the groin of an obese patient. The common sites are the inguinal and femoral, the inguinal immediately medial to the pubic tubercle and the femoral immediately lateral to it. The operation is naturally directed at the hernia in the first instance, although it may be necessary to open the general peritoneal cavity in order to facilitate the excision of a necrotic loop of bowel and the subsequent anastomosis.

Postoperative adhesions
The scars of surgical incisions on the anterior abdominal wall strongly suggest

that the cause of the intestinal obstruction is peritoneal adhesions. One or more loops of bowel becomes kinked by an adhesion between the loop and a fixed structure such as the scar on the inner aspect of the abdominal wall. Efficient nasogastric aspiration can reduce the pressure proximal to the obstruction, thereby facilitating unkinking of the loop and possibly relieving the obstruction. Experience teaches that it is worth trying the effect of conservative management in this group of cases for at least a few hours.

Pyloric outlet obstruction
This occurs in congenital and acquired forms.
Congenital   The presentation is usually in an infant between the ages of 4 weeks and 6 months, males being predominantly affected. The cause of the obstruction is a hypertrophy of the muscle of the antrum. The main symptom is vomiting immediately after eating, characteristically projectile in nature. The diagnosis is made by examining the infant during and immediately after its meal, when the ovoid swelling in the epigastrium becomes palpable. Mild cases may respond to treatment with inhibitors of the parasympathetic system (e.g. atropine methonitrate, Eumydrin), but in general the treatment after resuscitation is *Rammstedt's operation*: a longitudinal incision is made through the peritoneal covering and the muscle of the 'tumour', and deepened right down to the mucosa so that the two halves of the muscle fall apart. Any inadvertent incision into the mucosa itself must be carefully repaired. The results are excellent: this is one of the most immediately and completely effective operations in surgery.

Rarely, congenital hypertrophic pyloric stenosis may be encountered in an adult. It is usually misdiagnosed as a carcinoma of the antral region.
Acquired   Pyloric outflow obstruction in adults is usually due to stenosis of the first part of the duodenum in response to spasm and scarring from duodenal ulceration, or else to a carcinoma of the antrum. A typical peptic ulcer history over the previous month or years makes the the former diagnosis more likely, but otherwise the clinical features are almost identical. The cardinal symptom is vomiting, characteristically occurring at times remote from the last meal, very large in amount (more than 0.5 litre) and containing recognizable food that may have been eaten more than one meal previously (e.g. tomato pips, grape skins). The typical signs include visible peristalsis from left to right along the greater curvature of the grossly enlarged stomach, the succussion splash when the patient's trunk is shaken gently from side to side, and signs of extracellular depletion. Liquid aspirated from the stomach tends to be more acidic if the cause is duodenal ulcer than if the cause is carcinoma of the stomach, and correspondingly the metabolic alkalosis in patients with duodenal ulcer is more pronounced than in patients with carcinoma.

With this clinical picture there is no necessity to confirm the diagnosis with a barium meal; indeed, this investigation is contraindicated since the barium is likely to set into a solid mass with the retained food residues in the stomach and it then becomes very difficult to clean out the stomach. Gastroscopy and biopsy may yield the diagnosis but, because of the difficulty in cleaning out the stomach, this investigation often fails.

Management consists of preparing the stomach by washing it out, using in the first instance a wide-bore oesophageal tube if necessary because of the particulate debris blocking an ordinary nasogastric tube, followed by laparotomy. If the cause is a duodenal ulcer, some form of acid-reduction operation will be performed, and if this is a vagotomy then some drainage procedure must be added. Most surgeons do a gastroenterostomy or (if not technically too difficult) a pyloroplasty, while a few rely on dilating the stricture. Carcinoma of the stomach is treated if possible by gastrectomy (p. 40).

Gallstone ileus

A rare cause of intestinal obstruction which can occasionally be suspected before operation is obstruction due to the lodgement of a large gallstone in the ileum. Such a gallstone must have gained access to the alimentary tract via a fistula between the gall bladder and the duodenum, and the stone is likely to impact at the narrowest point of the bowel—which is usually in the terminal reaches of the ileum. En route to this point, the stone characteristically provokes a series of minor attacks of obstruction as it partially lodges here and there along the small bowel. The combination of a past history suggestive of gall bladder disease plus a series of such minor attacks of obstruction culminating in a complete small bowel obstruction suggests this diagnosis. At laparotomy the stone can often be crushed by pressure through the bowel wall and the fragments milked down into the large bowel. Occasionally an enterotomy is necessary.

Intussusception

This word signifies the telescoping of one portion of bowel into another; it results in strangulation-obstruction because the vessels in the mesentery of the ensheathed bit of bowel are compressed by the ensheathing portion of the bowel. Intussusception usually occurs in the prograde direction (i.e. in the direction of peristalsis), but very occasionally retrograde telescoping has been reported.

The common presentation is in infants around the age of 9–15 months, who suddenly become pale, scream with obvious abdominal pain, and pass a semi-liquid motion which is said to look like redcurrant jelly. This motion is mainly the mucus resulting from intestinal irritation, coloured by the dark plum-coloured venous bleeding produced by strangulation.

A barium enema examination confirms the diagnosis, and can be used with carefully regulated pressure of the introduced barium to attempt retrograde reduction of the intussusception. Should this technique fail, laparotomy is necessary to reduce the intussusception, if possible; alternatively, if the intussuscepted bowel is gangrenous, the lesion is resected and continuity restored by immediate anastomosis.

The cause of intussusception in childhood is unknown, although the fact that the usual site is the terminal ileum intussuscepting into the caecum and ascending colon has suggested that hypertrophy of the large Peyer's patches of lymphatic tissue in the terminal ileum initiate the intussusception. The condition can also occur in adults, but then there is nearly always an obvious cause for the invagination at the apex of the intussusception, often a benign and occasionally a malignant tumour projecting into the lumen from the wall of the bowel.

Volvulus of sigmoid

Volvulus is a condition in which part or all of an organ twists on its vascular pedicle; in this case, a loop of sigmoid colon twists on its mesentery, producing acute large bowel obstruction. There may be lesser premonitory attacks, but the established condition causes gross abdominal distension chiefly due to trapped flatus. The longer the sigmoid colon and the shorter the attachment of the sigmoid mesentery to the posterior abdominal wall, the greater the chance of volvulus. Racial and dietary factors may be important: volvulus is particularly common in Negroes and in people whose diet contains much poorly absorbable carbohydrates. Since these two factors coexist in many parts of Central Africa, the relative weight of each has not been worked out.

Volvulus occurs most often in middle-aged or elderly males: on examination the grossly distended abdomen yields a tympanitic percussion note, pain and tenderness are diffuse but may be most marked in the caecal region, and the appearances of plain x-ray are typically of a grossly distended sigmoid loop. Uncomplicated volvulus is amenable to non-operative treatment: a sigmoidoscope is passed and used to thread a large soft rubber tube into the sigmoid. If this manoeuvre is successful, the twisted loop deflates through the tube. At a later date it is wise to perform a laparotomy and excise the redundant loop of sigmoid because subsequent attacks are very common. Sigmoid colectomy might be necessary in the acute stage if deflation fails, and the Paul–Mikulicz operation (p. 114) is convenient.

The real problem is to recognize those patients in whom strangulation has been produced as well as intestinal obstruction. Rebound tenderness is not of much value because this sign can be obtained in any condition with dilated bowel; the important signs appear to be shock in excess of the degree that might be expected and absence of bowel sounds. Such evidence calls for immediate laparotomy, and a sigmoid resection with the formation of a Paul–Mikulicz type of double-barrelled colostomy is often the best operation.

Left-sided large bowel obstruction

This is a very common presentation of intestinal obstruction. The patients are usually middle-aged or elderly, and male. A history of change in bowel habit and, very likely, of blood in the motions is usually obtained, and the important clinical features of the final acute presentation include distension and absolute constipation with less emphasis on colicky abdominal pain, nausea and vomiting.

The most important condition causing left-sided bowel obstruction is carcinoma of the colon or rectum. About one-half of all carcinomas of the large bowel occur in the rectum or sigmoid and are therefore within the reach of a sigmoidoscope. This investigation is therefore mandatory at an early stage in the management of such patients. The other common cause is *diverticular disease of the colon*.

Carcinoma of the colon and rectum   Adenocarcinoma of the colon and rectum is one of the commonest cancers. In the Western world it is about as common as cancer of the stomach, and slightly less common than cancer of the bronchus and (in women) cancer of the breast. Despite all the improvements in medical and surgical care of the last three or four decades, there is no evidence that treatment of this condition has improved during that period. There are some well recognized specific aetiological factors: patients with *ulcerative colitis* show a strong tendency to develop malignant change when total colonic disease has been present for 10 years; patients with *familial polyposis of the colon*, a condition in which the whole of the large bowel is studded with innumerable small polyps, *always* develop cancer; however, individual solitary colonic polyps, more common on the left side of the bowel than the right, are very likely to become malignant if they increase in size to a diameter greater than 2 cm. There is also increasing evidence that some dietary factor is involved in the aetiology of those cases in which the specific factors are absent. There seems to be a link between a high intake of calories—independent of fish and of fat—and the incidence of colorectal cancer, while a lack of bran in the diet also may be a risk factor.

Carcinoma of the colon in its common sites in the left half of the colon, especially the rectosigmoid region, is likely to present with obstruction, whereas in the caecum and transverse colon where the contents of bowel are liquid and considerable bleeding from an ulcerated lesion can occur without overt evidence in the stools, the common presentation is chronic iron-deficiency anaemia.

Diverticular disease of the colon   For further information about this condition, see p. 113.

The basic cause is unknown, but it has been demonstrated that in many cases of diverticular disease with symptoms there is a higher pressure than average within the lumen of the rectosigmoid region. This fact, taken in conjunction with the evidence that diverticulosis, while undeniably often symptomless, is often associated with constipation and the passage of small hard stools, has led to the suggestion that people with symptoms should be treated with a high residue diet (i.e. bran).

Apart from chronic constipation, sometimes alternating with diarrhoea so that the possibility of a colonic neoplasm is raised, diverticular disease can give rise to a number of complications: infection with the formation of a pericolic abscess and possible perforation into the peritoneal cavity producing peritonitis (p. 113); severe rectal haemorrhage (p. 128); and intestinal obstruction due to spasm and kinking by adhesions. The distinction from left-sided obstruction due to carcinoma can be very difficult to make, and indeed it may not be possible to decide until laparotomy and biopsy whether the colonic mass is entirely inflammatory or partly neoplastic. In particular, it is important not to accept radiological evidence of diverticulosis as implying that the cause of the obstruction is diverticular disease: remember the very common occurrence of diverticulosis!

Bleeding from the alimentary tract

Bleeding from the alimentary tract may result from trauma, but this section is concerned with haemorrhage resulting from gastrointestinal disease. The bleeding may become manifest at either the upper or the lower end of the alimentary tract. When the blood is vomited, the condition is called *haematemesis*. When blood altered by the processes of digestion appears at the anal canal as a black tarry liquid, the term *melaena* is used. In practice it can be accepted that haematemesis means the blood has come from a lesion proximal to the duodenojejunal junction, while melaena means that the blood has been shed at some point well proximal to the colon so that there has been time for some of the processes of digestion to occur. Lesions which give rise to haematemesis may also give rise to melaena, and melaena may also occur in lesions of the proximal half or so of the small bowel. Rectal haemorrhage usually comes from a lesion of the large bowel, but it is important to appreciate that very rapid bleeding from the proximal bowel may result in such a rapid transit along the intestinal tract that the blood emerges unchanged at the anus. Thus there are two separate presentations—haematemesis and/or melaena on the one hand, and rectal haemorrhage on the other.

Haematemesis and melaena

The principles of management are to resuscitate the patient, to determine the cause of the bleeding and to do whatever is indicated to stop the bleeding. If the patient has bled heavily and is in severe shock by the time he is seen by the clinician, the first priority is to save life and this means the setting up of an intravenous infusion to restore the blood volume by crystalloid or plasma or plasma substitute, and later, when it becomes available, fully cross-matched blood. When the patient's condition has stabilized, or in patients with less severe bleeding right from the onset, attempts to diagnose the cause can begin.

In England and Wales there are about 20 000 hospital admissions each year with acute haematemesis and melaena. The common causes are chronic peptic ulcers of the stomach or duodenum, acute erosions or stress ulcers, a Mallory–Weiss tear and peptic oesophagitis. Uncommon lesions include oesophagogastric varices in patients with portal hypertension, and tumours of the oesophagus and stomach, usually malignant. Much rarer are bleeding disorders, angiomatous malformations, aortic aneurysm (eroding through into the duodenum) and excessive anticoagulant treatment.

A history of chronic indigestion suggestive of peptic ulceration or of alcoholism can be significant. Similarly, an upper abdominal palpable mass may suggest carcinoma of the stomach, while the stigmata of hepatic failure suggest portal hypertension. Certain drugs such as salicylates, corticosteroids and indomethacin are known to increase the chance of bleeding from chronic peptic ulcers, while any severely ill patient (from whatever cause, be it severe burns, multiple trauma or overwhelming septicaemia) is liable to stress ulceration of the stomach and duodenum—a poorly understood condition in which haemorrhagic inflammation or multiple shallow ulcers develop in the gastric or duodenal mucosa.

Conventional history and examination suggest a cause of bleeding in about half the cases, but the suggestion is often incorrect. For example, haematemesis and melaena in patients with proven portal hypertension are more likely to be from peptic ulceration than from varices. Thus more reliable methods of diagnosis are essential.

The method of choice is oesophagogastroduodenoscopy, carried out 12–48 hours after admission when the patient's condition is stable. Blood in the stomach may obscure bleeding sites, but an accurate diagnosis can usually be obtained. If endoscopy fails, or is contraindicated or not available, then it is worth getting an upper gastrointestinal opaque meal x-ray examination; this will probably reveal such lesions as a chronic peptic ulcer or oesophageal varices, but will almost certainly not pick up surface lesions such as shallow erosions.

If endoscopy and opaque meal radiology are both unsuccessful, it is necessary to look for rare causes of bleeding such as blood dyscrasias and angiomas. In the diagnosis of the latter, x-ray angiography during the bleed may demonstrate the lesions. Angiomatous malformations may occur anywhere in the mucosa of the alimentary tract, and can be very difficult to diagnose.

When the cause has been determined, a logical plan of treatment can be constructed.

Chronic peptic ulcer
In the first instance, treatment is expectant. If the patient has been on drugs known to be associated with haematemesis, these are stopped and it is usually advised that cimetidine be started. The evidence suggests that cimetidine is not of much value in the treatment of haemorrhage from a chronic peptic ulcer, but lowering gastric acid production with full doses of cimetidine (p. 57) does seem to be valuable in the management of stress ulceration. Persistent or torrential bleeding or recurrence during the same admission are indications for operation, and this is particularly true the older the patient. Certain features of the endoscopic examination are also recognized as indicating that a local blood vessel is very likely to bleed again; for example, a blood clot adherent to the mucosa or black slough in the base of an ulcer.

The principles of the operation are some form of attack upon the ulcer itself to prevent acute bleeding, together with some form of acid reduction procedure to prevent recurrence of the ulcer. For duodenal ulceration, many surgeons under-run the crater with non-absorbable sutures to obliterate the feeding vessel and perform a vagotomy, usually with drainage, while for gastric ulcer the most common form of treatment is a partial gastrectomy, as part of which the ulcer itself is removed.

Mallory–Weiss tear
Protracted vomiting induces one or more linear tears in the mucosa at the gastro-oesophageal junction. The amount of bleeding is usually not very great and active treatment is rarely indicated.

Oesophageal varices

This is one of the most important complications of portal hypertension (Chapter 6). While comparatively uncommon in the United Kingdom, it is a much more important cause of haematemesis and melaena in countries with a larger incidence of chronic alcoholism. The routine management is with a Blakemore–Sengstaken tube. This is a soft tube which is swallowed so that its tip lies in the stomach; it has two balloons, one lying within the stomach and the other in the region of the lower third of the oesophagus. Each balloon can be separately inflated: the lower balloon keeps the tip of the tube within the stomach while the upper exerts pressure on the oesophageal varices. The stomach contents can be aspirated through the main channel from the tip, and oesophageal secretions from extra holes above the oesophageal balloon; this last precaution reduces the chance of aspiration pneumonia. The oesophageal pressure must be released at intervals to prevent pressure necrosis. In addition to, or instead of, this tube, conservative management can include the injection of vasopressin (Pitressin) 20 units in 100 ml 5 per cent dextrose given intravenously over the course of 15 minutes; this agent is effective in reducing the pressure in the portal venous system. Portacaval shunts to decompress the portal-venous system are not usually recommended as an emergency measure for bleeding oesophageal varices. Other operations attack the varices themselves; for example, ligating them through the wall of the lower oesophagus or transecting the oesophagogastric junction and then reanastomosing (Tanner's operation). These major procedures requiring laparotomy or laparotomy and thoracotomy carry a heavy mortality, although modern automatic stapling devices (the 'gun') have facilitated the technicalities, and the emphasis at present is on other techniques for obliterating the varices: by the injection of sclerosant material via an endoscope or by embolizing them through their main supplying vein with material such as fibrin or gelatin foam (Gelfoam): this material is introduced into the vein via a transhepatic catheter and the portal venous system. The emboli lodge in the varices, promoting a marked tissue reaction which culminates in fibrosis and obliteration of the varices. This is a very difficult field, as demonstrated by the large number of methods of treatment.

Other lesions found by endoscopy are treated on their merits. If no lesion can be demonstrated but the bleeding becomes very severe, 'blind' laparotomy may be necessary but most surgeons would agree that this procedure is seldom rewarding.

Rectal haemorrhage

Rapid rectal bleeding should always be treated conservatively in the first instance because it is usually self-limiting. Having restored the blood loss by transfusion if necessary, and waited for the bleeding to stop, investigation proceeds along the usual lines for large bowel disease—sigmoidoscopy, barium enema and possibly colonoscopy.

Until recently it was thought that the major cause of rapid rectal haemorrhage was diverticular disease. This idea was fostered by the common finding of diverticulosis in barium enema examinations (p. 113). In consequence, many patients underwent resection of the left side of the colon and afterwards continued to have rectal bleeding! The most common source of bleeding from the colon is an angiomatous malformation in the *right* half. Important aids to diagnosis are colonoscopy and radiological angiography with the selective injection of contrast material into the superior mesenteric and inferior mesenteric arteries. When such malformations occur in the small bowel they are beyond the reach of the colonoscope and thus exceedingly difficult to diagnose.

Severe bleeding may occur from any lesion of the large bowel such as carcinoma of the colon.

Massive diarrhoea

The copious liquid motions of a patient with severe diarrhoea approximate in composition to the extracellular fluid with the exception that the potassium ion concentration, approximately 18 mmol/l, is considerably higher than the 5 mmol/l of the extracellular space. Thus the pathophysiological consequences of the diarrhoea are, first and foremost, a contraction of the extracellular volume with a corresponding haemoconcentration and fall in the circulating blood volume, and, secondly, when the diarrhoea has been present for some time, hypokalaemia. Accordingly, the first consideration in resuscitation is to replenish the extracellular space and thus the plasma volume with normal saline or similar solutions, and when urinary output has increased to reasonable levels to add potassium.

Patients with acute massive diarrhoea may have other symptoms and signs such as griping abdominal pain, nausea and vomiting. Diagnosis may be aided by features in the history or the examination, but the definitive investigations are cultures of the blood and stools, the appearances on sigmoidoscopy, the microscopic appearance of biopsies of the rectal mucosa, the culture of scrapings obtained at sigmoidoscopy, and finally specific tests for the diseases which can cause this fulminating picture.

Cholera

This disease is produced by *Vibrio cholerae*, a Gram-negative comma-shaped organism. The main endemic centre of this disease is Bangladesh, whence epidemics spread to many other parts of the world.

Cholera produces a toxin which acts by increasing adenyl cyclase activity in the cells lining the small bowel. This results in an increase in synthesis of cyclic AMP, which causes a huge secretion of chloride into the lumen (Sanford: *Digestive System Physiology*, Chapter 5). Sodium and water move with the chloride, while potassium is present at a concentration of about 18 mmol/l (18 mEq/l) in all secretions of the alimentary tract (except saliva). The stools are almost clear water with flecks of mucus and look rather like the water in which rice is boiled ('rice-water stools').

The diagnosis can be confirmed bacteriologically, and the treatment, apart from restoration of the extracellular fluid, is tetracycline. In any case, the disease is self-limiting in about 3 days provided that the patient is kept alive by adequate fluid and electrolyte therapy during that time.

'Antibiotic-associated colitis'

Very severe forms of enterocolitis with diarrhoea occur in patients who have been on oral antibiotic treatment. It would appear that these cases are due to a disturbance of the normal balance of fauna in the bowel and the emergence of strains which are usually present only in small quantities.

The commonest organism to produce this syndrome until recently was the *Staphylococcus*, and this was best diagnosed by immediate Gram-staining and microscopic examination of scrapings from the wall of the rectum obtained via the sigmoidoscope. More recently, an anaerobic organism called *Clostridium difficile* has been found in an increasing proportion of cases, usually in patients who have had lincomycin. It is said that patients with this particular condition show an appearance of membrane formation—the 'pseudomembrane'—over the surface of the rectal mucosa. However, this field is a new one and several points remain vague. The specific treatment sometimes recommended for *C. difficile* infections is metronidazole or vancomycin, but many clinicians feel that all antibiotics should be avoided because spontaneous recovery is the rule.

Other infections

Most of the other infective causes produce symptoms that are less acutely severe, although the occasional patient may present with fulminant diarrhoea. These recognized enteric infections include bacillary dysentery, *Salmonella* infections, amoebiasis and food poisoning.

Shigellosis (bacillary dysentery)

Shigellosis is an acute colitis produced by *Shigella* organisms, which are Gram-negative non-motile facultative anaerobic bacilli. There are four species of *Shigella* organisms: *dysenteriae, flexneri, boydii* and *sonnei*. Their distribution is world-wide, they are excreted in the faeces of individuals with symptoms and (rarely) by symptomless carriers, and transfer is usually via inadequately washed hands contaminated with faeces although passive transfer by flies is possible. Colicky abdominal pain, headache and fever may precede the diarrhoea for 1 or 2 days. The stools contain acute inflammatory cells, a characteristic shared with ulcerative colitis but with no other bowel disorders, and the organism can usually be cultured from the stools. Most strains are sensitive to ampicillin.

Salmonellosis

The Salmonellae are a complex group of organisms: they are Gram-negative rods and facultative anaerobes. There are many species, including the familiar *S. typhi* and the *S. paratyphi*. Clinical manifestations of infection may be confined to the alimentary tract (non-typhoidal salmonellosis) or there may be penetration of the organisms throughout the body, producing typhoid or the milder paratyphoid fever. Humans are usually infected by contaminated food, and there is evidence that the most frequent source of contamination is animal rather than human. Patients with the acute infection have positive stool cultures for 2–10 weeks after the symptoms have subsided, and treatment with antibiotics prolongs this period of symptomless excretion. The clinical picture is variable but essentially that of an acute febrile gastroenteritis.

Infection with *S. typhi* always results in clinical disease. There is a septicaemia with hyperplasia and focal necrosis in lymph nodes, bronchitis and pneumonia, occasionally mild cholecystitis, and local abscesses. The changes in the bowel can give rise to severe intestinal haemorrhage and/or perforation. The stools, as in other forms of bacillary dysentery, contain leucocytes and the organism can be grown from them. Throat swabs and blood cultures are also often positive, and there are characteristic agglutination reactions to help identify the organism.

The best agent for treating this condition is chloramphenicol, although ampicillin is also quite effective. The chronic carrier state, with patients excreting the organisms in their faeces for months or years after what might have been a mild attack, is not prevented by antibiotic treatment and may indeed be predisposed to by it because relapses are common after the antibiotic is stopped. The gall bladder is the common source of the organisms in the carrier state: cholecystectomy is advised for identified carriers.

Amoebiasis

Rarely, acute amoebic colitis can present with severe diarrhoea containing blood and mucus. The sigmoidoscopic appearances of multiple small ulcers containing yellow slough and set in a background of intense inflammation of the mucosa may be characteristic, but the diagnosis is made by examination of the stool for cysts and parasites (p. 76).

Food poisoning

The two important conditions under this heading that may produce severe diarrhoea are *botulism* and *staphylococcal* poisoning. Botulism is due to toxins produced by *Clostridium botulinum*; although symptoms and signs of a gastroenteritis may occur, the most important effects of the toxin are on the central nervous system where it has a curare-like action on the motor end-plate. The presence of the toxin in the blood can be confirmed by the appropriate serological test; the effects of the toxin are temporary, and the patient should recover if he can be kept alive by artificial ventilation during the stage of paralysis. Canned foods are the main source of this problem.

Staphylococcal poisoning due to the toxins produced by *Staphylococcus aureus* is a severe but brief disease with abdominal symptoms and prostration, but self-limiting and lasting only 12–24 hours. The outbreak typically affects a large number of people at the same time.

Ulcerative colitis

If the sigmoidoscopic appearances are those of a florid inflammation of the mucosa with loss of vascular pattern and a readiness to bleed on contact with the sigmoidoscope, and if no pathogens are isolated from the stools, then the conclusion must be that the patient is suffering from ulcerative colitis of which one form is a fulminant attack of very sudden onset without any previous history suggestive of large bowel disease. This condition is considered in more detail on p. 144.

Further reading

British Journal of Hospital Medicine (1980). Symposium on gastrointestinal bleeding. **23**, 333–365.

Cohen, M. M. (1971). Treatment and mortality of perforated peptic ulcer: a survey of 852 cases. *Canadian Medical Association Journal* **105**, 263–269.

Cope, Z. (1979). *The Early Diagnosis of the Acute Abdomen.* Oxford University Press, Oxford.

Dunphy, J. E. (1981). The acute abdomen. In *Current Surgical Diagnosis and Treatment,* 5th edition pp. 385–394. Ed. by J. E. Dunphy and L. W. Way. Lange, Los Altos, California.

Greenberger, N. J., Arvanitakis, C. and Hurwitz, A. (1979). *Drug Treatment of Intestinal Disorders.* Churchill Livingstone, Edinburgh.

Howat, H. T. and Sarles, H. (1979). *The Exocrine Pancreas.* W. B. Saunders, London, Philadelphia and Toronto.

Le Quesne, L. P. (1976). Acute intestinal obstruction. In *Current Surgical Practice,* vol. 1, pp. 168–184. Ed. by G. J. Hadfield and M. Hobsley. Edward Arnold, London.

Morson, B. C. and Dawson, I. M. P. (1972). *Gastrointestinal Pathology.* Blackwell Scientific, Oxford.

Nixon, H. H. (1976). Intestinal obstruction in the newborn. In *Current Surgical Practice,* vol. 1, pp. 149–167. Ed. by G. J. Hadfield and M. Hobsley. Edward Arnold, London.

Robarts, W. M. Parkin, J. V. and Hobsley, M. (1979). A simple clinical approach to quantifying losses from the extracellular and plasma compartments. *Annals of the Royal College of Surgeons of England* **61**, 142–145.

Shields, R. (1965). The absorption and secretion of fluid and electrolytes by the obstructed bowel. *British Journal of Surgery* **52**, 774–779.

Smith, A. N. (Ed.) (1975). *Diverticular Disease. Clinics in Gastroenterology* **4**, no. 1.

Taha, S. E. and Suleiman, S. I. (1980). Volvulus of the sigmoid colon in the Gezira. *British Journal of Surgery* **67**, 433–435.

Trapnell, J. E. (1976). Pancreatitis: acute and chronic. In *Current Surgical Practice,* vol. 1, pp. 132–148. Ed. by G. J. Hadfield and M. Hobsley. Edward Arnold, London.

Trewby, P. N. (1980). Drug-induced peptic ulcer and upper gastrointestinal bleeding. *British Journal of Hospital Medicine* **23**, 185–190.

Van der Linden, W. and Sunzel, H. (1970). Early versus delayed operation for acute cholecystitis: a controlled clinical trial. *American Journal of Surgery* **120**, 7–13.

Wilson, J. P. (1975). Postoperative motility of the large intestine in man. *Gut* **16**, 689–692.

8

Disturbances of defaecation

A change in bowel habit often signals serious disease and should therefore always be taken seriously.

History

Normal bowel habit

Bowel habit has a wide range of normality. One should (in the United Kingdom) accept as normal any frequency in the range once every third day to three times daily, but the exact limits vary in other parts of the world, doubtless due to racial as well as environmental considerations such as nature of the food eaten, and habit and custom. It is important to take a careful drug history. Laxative abuse is common, and many drugs besides the obvious example of opiates (e.g. anti-hypertensive agents, antacids and antidepressives) affect bowel motility. It is also important to enquire about the habitual consistency of the patient's motions, because this can vary from liquid to hard solid and still be the norm for that individual. Indeed, not everyone is privileged to pass one soft, but formed, motion daily!

Chronic change in bowel habit

In this chapter we consider only chronic disturbances; acute diarrhoea, constipation and bleeding are considered in Chapter 7. Thus the changes are not so severe as to force the patient to seek medical advice within hours or a few days of their onset—although pain on defaecation can be an exception.

Types of change
Diarrhoea is a symptom variably defined by different authorities. Certainly a motion that is more liquid than the patient's norm constitutes diarrhoea: the problem is whether a *frequency* of defaecation greater than normal also, in itself, does. My tendency is to place more reliance on consistency than frequency. Chronic diarrhoeic motions are usually paler than normal, but retain some faecal coloration, unlike the colourless rice-water stools of the acute diarrhoeas such as cholera (Chapter 7).

Steatorrhoea is a special form of diarrhoea in which the motion looks greasy and very pale in colour and floats on water. These appearances are due to undigested and unabsorbed fat, and because such stools are associated with rapid transit they often contain undigested protein (e.g. muscle fibres) of the ingested food.

Constipation means difficulty in passing a motion due to its hardness. A reduction in frequency of defaecation should not in itself be called constipation if the motion is passed easily and without straining. Notice that by this definition many individuals are *normally* constipated; it is an *increase* in difficulty that alerts the clinician.

Alternating constipation and diarrhoea is a particularly important feature because it is typical of incomplete large bowel obstruction due to a colonic tumour. A carcinoma half fills the lumen of the left side of the colon; a lump of solid faeces impacts temporarily and constipation ensues. The obstruction of the colon and the presence of the tumour both irritate the colon, which responds by its usual reaction of secreting mucus and extracellular fluid containing bicarbonate. Most of these secretions are dammed up behind the obstruction. Then, by chance, the obstructing faecal pellet is dislodged and there is a gush of faeces and secretions into the rectum, resulting in urgency and diarrhoea.

The passage of mucus by itself is strongly suggestive of an irritant lesion of the lower colon. Typical causes include a pelvic abscess, carcinoma of the rectosigmoid and a villous adenoma of the rectosigmoid, but it can also occur in the functional disorder known as 'irritable bowel' or indeed 'mucous colitis'.

The passage of blood is a crucially important complaint, not only because it is so often due to a serious cause but also because its characteristics can point to the cause. Leaving aside frank melaena and massive haemorrhage (Chapter 7), blood passed per anum is either always associated with the act of defaecation or else occurs separately from defaecation as well, it may be described as bright or dark in colour, and either is well mixed with the faeces or is passed as a separate coating on the surface of the stool or on the lavatory pan or the toilet paper shortly after defaecation. Blood at times other than defaecation probably arises in an ulcerative lesion such as a carcinoma. Bright blood has been very recently shed and probably has arisen in an anal lesion such as haemorrhoids or a fissure, while dark blood has probably originated higher up the bowel, especially if it has mixed in well with the stool. A spurt of bright red blood into the pan immediately · after defaecation is typical of haemorrhoids or a fissure.

The passage of a mixture of pure blood and mucus suggests an acutely irritant and ulcerative lesion; i.e. a colitis such as ulcerative, Crohn's or amoebic colitis.

Pain is also helpful. Pain on defaecation only rarely occurs with lesions of the rectum or colon: it is a result of anal or perianal pathology. Haemorrhoids are not usually painful unless strangulated, although they become tender if they are chronically prolapsed and the patient is having to sit on them. However, a fissure is exquisitely painful during, and for minutes or hours after, the act of defaecation. Longer lasting pain is due to strangulated piles or a perianal haematoma. Nocturnal attacks of anal pain—severe but self-limiting after minutes or hours and lacking physical signs—are called *proctalgia fugax*; their aetiology is unknown.

Prolapse, the complaint that something 'comes down' on defaecation that is not faeces is usually indicative of haemorrhoids but the prolapsing material may occasionally be a tumour—benign or malignant—of the rectum.

Tenesmus is the sensation of something stuck in the anal canal that does not move on if defaecation is attempted or achieved. The sensation is usually produced by a carcinoma of the lower rectum or the anal canal itself.

Finally, *urgency* and *incontinence* are self-explanatory. *True incontinence* results from inefficiency of the anal sphincter due to local destructive lesions—inflammatory or neoplastic—to diseases of the nervous controlling mechanisms, or to inherent failure of the sphincter musculature (lack in tone) as in old age. *Overflow incontinence* is the leakage of faecally stained mucus around a mass of hard faeces (scybala) impacted in the rectum and anal canal.

Physical signs

This section concentrates on signs in the abdomen, including the rectum and anal canal, and in the perineum. Diseases causing disturbances of defaecation may produce generalized or systemic signs such as anaemia, weight loss and evidence of deficiency of vitamins. Such general manifestations are considered later (with malabsorption).

Abdomen

Distension means an *increase* in tension within the abdominal cavity; on attempting to deform the abdominal wall the observer meets resistance greater than he would expect. Thus this physical sign relies greatly on the ability of the patient to relax his abdominal musculature. A good objective guide is eversion of the umbilicus, provided that the patient is sure that the eversion is not normally present.

Distension is due to the accumulation within the abdomen of *gas* in the intestines, or of *liquid* in the peritoneal cavity, or to a very large *tumour*. Gas is resonant on percussion; its presence suggests intestinal obstruction, particularly of the large bowel variety (Chapter 7), but it is common in flatulent dyspepsia (Chapter 3). Liquid, i.e. *ascites* (Chapter 6), is dull to percussion. A large tumour producing distension originates usually in the reproductive system (gravid uterus or ovarian cyst) but occasionally in the gastrointestinal tract.

Visible peristalsis indicates that the stomach or bowel is vigorously attempting to overcome a partial obstruction.

A *loaded sigmoid colon* may be palpable in the left iliac fossa. The mass of faeces may be surprisingly hard, but its nature is indicated by its indentability when pressed with the tip of a finger. This sign implies constipation, and it is particularly useful if the patient is complaining of diarrhoea which can then be adjudged to be spurious.

Other evidence of particular intra-abdominal lesions may of course be obtained, including masses, especially a palpable liver, ascites and abnormalities on auscultation.

Rectal examination

Inspection
This includes the anus, its immediate surroundings and the whole of the perineum, the sacral region and the buttocks; i.e. all those parts which are not very easily examined except in the left lateral or lithotomy positions.

Pilonidal sinus   The solitary, or more typically multiple, pinpoint openings of this lesion are characteristically visible in the upper part of the natal cleft, 5–15 cm above the anus (Fig. 8.1a). If active infection of the lesion is present, there is a tender area of redness and induration in or near the midline in the vicinity of these openings, and sometimes the openings themselves are no longer visible because of obliteration by oedema. Pilonidal sinus is an acquired lesion, resulting from the penetration of loose hairs through the skin of the natal cleft. *Pilonidal* means 'a nest of hairs', and sometimes the cavity deep to the skin contains a mass of the patient's hair. Superadded infection results in an abscess.

The features predisposing to a pilonidal sinus are hairiness, especially in association with black wiry hair, and maceration of the skin of the region with sweat, especially with minor trauma; hence it was common in soldiers driving in jeeps over the uneven terrain of the Western Desert in the Second World War ('jeep disease').

Treatment follows standard surgical lines of incision and drainage, opening up the whole abscess cavity to free drainage. Some surgeons advise wide excision but this necessitates a complicated repair and does not guarantee freedom from recurrence. For unknown reasons, recurrences, although common in young adults, are rare once the age of about 40 years is reached and so minimal treatment such as incision and drainage is preferable to complicated operations.

'Piles'   This is a layman's term used to describe any lump presenting at the anal verge. Common lesions visible at the anal verge include skin tags (also called external piles), the so-called 'sentinel pile' which is a prominent skin tag at the lower end of an anal fissure, usually in the midline posteriorly but in women sometimes in the midline anteriorly, and anal warts which are common multiple and filiform, and are one form of venereal disease. A *fissure* itself (Fig. 8.1b) cannot usually be seen, but its presence may be suspected from tight spasm of the sphincter ani producing a corrugated appearance of the external orifice in combination with a sentinel pile. A *thrombosed external pile* is a very acutely painful swelling due to rupture of a subcutaneous vessel at the anal verge, leading to a tense haematoma. The condition is self-limiting, but in the acute phase a small local incision to evacuate the clot under local anaesthesia provides excellent relief. *Prolapse* of anal mucosa may be immediately visible (Fig. 8.1c) or may only become so when the patient is asked to strain down. The segmental prolapse of internal haemorrhoids (Fig. 8.1d) can be readily distinguished from circumferential prolapse but the latter

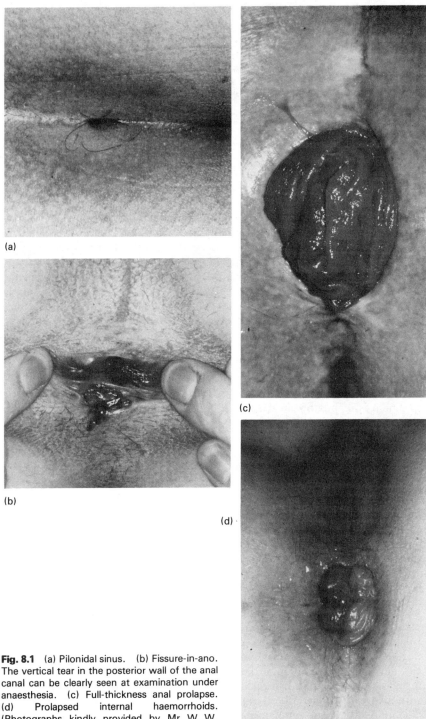

(a)

(b)

(c)

(d)

Fig. 8.1 (a) Pilonidal sinus. (b) Fissure-in-ano. The vertical tear in the posterior wall of the anal canal can be clearly seen at examination under anaesthesia. (c) Full-thickness anal prolapse. (d) Prolapsed internal haemorrhoids. (Photographs kindly provided by Mr W. W. Slack)

may be full-thickness or just a prolapse of the anal mucosa, these two possibilities can be distinguished by palpation.

Fistula-in-ano   This presents as one or more opening on the surface of the skin in the perianal region. A symmetrical opening on each side in the posterior half of the perianal region is often encountered and the two tracks commonly unite in the midline behind the anus, to form a complete fistula with the lumen of the anus via a single posterior track. Fistulae in this situation are due primarily to infection with pus formation in lymph glands in the wall of the anal canal, the pus tracking both into the anal cavity and via the perianal tissues to the skin surface. Sometimes pus accumulates in the deep fibrofatty space of the ischiorectal fossa lateral to the anal canal and lower rectum, and this presents as an *ischiorectal abscess* with a painful tender induration to one or other side of the anal canal. An abscess must be deroofed to provide adequate drainage; when the acute inflammation has subsided, the abscess cavity is reviewed under anaesthesia to determine whether there is a fistulous track into the anal canal. Such a fistulous track must be laid open completely by passing a pliable metal director along the track and cutting down upon it from the exterior; with really adequate drainage like this the lesion heals. A particularly difficult problem requiring highly expert management is the so-called *high fistula* in which the track lies above the musculature of the anal sphincters: laying open such a track would carry the danger of incompetence at the anus.

Ulcers   Ulcers at the anus or perianal region may be painless or painful. Painless ulcers suggest syphilis, Crohn's disease or carcinoma, while painful ulcers may be due to herpes, a condition which in some parts of the world is the most common venereal disease! Histological examination of a biopsy specimen is mandatory in the management of ulcers. This statement is true also of non-ulcerated masses which are not readily recognizable.

Palpation

The most important aspect of digital examination is whether one can feel a mass within the anus or rectum, the most likely diagnosis of such a mass being carcinoma. The laxity or normality of the external sphincter should also be noted—this aspect being important in the diagnosis of faecal incontinence—and a fissure diagnosed by marked tenderness in the midline posteriorly in both sexes (or, in women, anteriorly); this tenderness usually prevents further examination. Acute fissures like this should be treated by giving the patient an anal dilator to be smeared liberally with a local anaesthetic such as lignocaine gel and passed twice daily including before defaecation. An anal fissure is a longitudinal slit in the anal mucosa, usually produced by straining to pass a hard stool; the pain results in anal spasm which, due to the circumferential arrangement of the fibres of the external sphincter, pulls the edges of the fissure apart and prevents healing. Breaking this vicious circle with topical analgesia usually permits healing to occur. A chronic fissure is readily palpable as a mass of fibrous tissue arranged linearly in the anal canal; such fissures, together with acute fissures that fail to heal with the treatment described, require an operation under anaesthetic—simple dilatation of the anal canal, or an operation to divide the external sphincter or a complete fissurectomy.

Internal haemorrhoids are *not* palpable. A *polyp*, i.e. any pedunculated lesion of the lower rectum or anal canal, may be palpable.

Proctoscopy

Inspection of the anal canal with a lighted speculum called a proctoscope or anoscope, reaching to the level of the anorectal ring, reveals *internal haemorrhoids*. These lesions are segmentally arranged redundancies of the anal mucosa with a tendency to prolapse and bleed. The prolapsing masses commonly lie at 3 o'clock, 8 o'clock and 10 o'clock (as one looks at the patient in the lithotomy position), and because these positions corrrespond with the arrangement of the inferior rectal vessels into two right lateral and one left lateral vessel, internal haemorrhoids have in the past been described as dilatations of the veins of the inferior haemorrhoidal plexus. Even the term *varicosity* has been used, but this is absurd since a varicose vein by definition is one with incompetent valves and there are no valves in the haemorrhoidal plexus of veins.

Internal haemorrhoids bleed bright red blood when traumatized by the passage of hard faeces, the submucosal tissue being a pulp of very rich arteriovenous connections resembling the erectile tissue of the corpora cavernosa of the penis. Bleeding occurs with and after defaecation, and is particularly severe if prolapse is marked so that the patient is constantly sitting upon his piles and abrading their surface.

First degree piles do not prolapse. They draw attention to themselves only by bleeding, and respond well (though not necessarily permanently) to injections of sclerosant material such as phenol dissolved in almond oil into the submucosal tissue at the leve of the anorectal ring. The resultant fibrosis draws up the redundant mucosa. Third degree piles which are perpetually prolapsed require operative treatment: the standard operation is called *haemorrhoidectomy*, but good results are also being obtained with the application of elastic bands to the pedicle of the pile which results in their thrombosis and sloughing. Second degree piles, which prolapse on straining but reduce themselves spontaneously, can be given a trial of injection therapy but if they cause considerable trouble require operative treatment by haemorrhoidectomy or forcible dilatation.

Polypoid lesions of the anal canal are noted at proctoscopy and are an indication for repeating the examination under anaesthesia and excising them for histological examination.

Sigmoidoscopy

This investigation can be performed as an outpatient procedure without anaesthesia; the rigid sigmoidoscope used in these circumstances is about 2 cm in diameter and 25 cm in length. The patient is placed in the left lateral, the lithotomy or the knee–elbow position. Under a general anaesthetic a large-bore sigmoidoscope can be passed to permit various manipulative procedures such as the snaring of a polyp. However, a biopsy can be taken painlessly via the outpatient type of sigmoidscope. Even experienced clinicians often find it difficult to negotiate the bend at the rectosigmoid junction, 10–12 cm from the anus. A flexible fibreoptic sigmoidoscope is now available.

The most important lesion that can be visualized with the sigmoidscope is carcinoma of the rectum or sigmoid: a substantial proportion of all carcinomas of the large bowel can be reached with the sigmoidoscope and biopsied. The naked eye appearance may be an ulcer with heaped-up edges, a cauliflower-like growth or a ring stricture. Apart from getting the specimen, the examination must establish how close to the anal margin the lesion extends (p. 142).

Other lesions that may be visualized include *polyps, villous adenoma,* the mouths of diverticula and inflammation of the rectal mucosa (i.e. proctitis). The appearances of ulcerative colitis and amoebic colitis have already been described (Chapter 7), while the villous adenoma is a multiple papillary lesion of glistening white appearance.

Examination of the faeces

In patients in whom the clinical circumstances suggest an attack of gastroenteritis or recurrent diarrhoea which might be associated with malabsorption (p. 148), specimens of the faeces are examined for pathogenic bacteria and parasites. This line of investigation also needs to be pursued in those patients in whom sigmoidoscopy, barium enema and, if performed, colonoscopy have proved negative (assuming that the symptoms persist).

Special investigations

Barium enema

Even when sigmoidoscopy has demonstrated a lesion that would explain the symptoms and other signs, barium enema must be performed. Multiple lesions are not very uncommon in the colon. About 2 per cent of all patients with a carcinoma of the colon have a second *synchronous* carcinoma somewhere else in the large bowel. This is not surprising when one remembers that *adenomatous polyps,* in which many carcinomas arise by malignant transformation, are multiple. The preparation of the bowel by suitable enemas and aperients is crucial to the success of a barium enema x-ray examination (Fig. 8.2).

Intravenous pyelogram

If an operation to excise the rectum is contemplated, many clinicians order an intravenous pyelogram to check the position of the ureters. The latter, especially the left, can easily be distorted by the presence of a carcinoma of the sigmoid and be at risk during the operation unless its bizarre course is known. Early warning of involvement of the ureter—which may mean that a length of ureter will have to be sacrificed and replaced or even that a nephrectomy is necessary—may also be demonstrated.

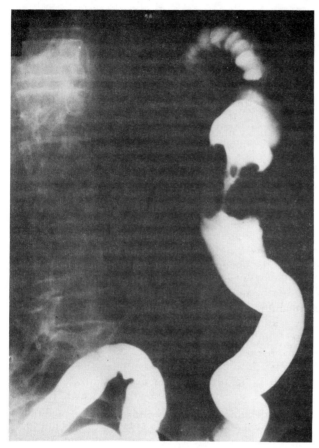

Fig. 8.2 Barium enema, showing a carcinoma of the descending colon. Prominent 'shoulders' at the two ends of the stricture represent the everted edges of a circumferential ulcer, and produce an 'apple-core' appearance.

Colonoscopy

With patience, an experienced colonoscopist can pass the instrument right round the large bowel to the caecum in more than 90 per cent of patients; in the others, a view considerably higher than that obtained with the conventional sigmoidoscopy can be gained. Colonoscopy is useful if there is a strong suspicion of a macroscopic lesion such as carcinoma or ulcerative colitis in the colon but sigmoidoscopy and barium enema have proved negative. Since the examination may take up to an hour of the patient's and the colonoscopist's time, it is not to be lightly undertaken! If a lesion is demonstrated biopsies can be taken, and pedunculated polyps can be removed by diathermy snare.

Diagnosis made

Carcinoma of the colon and rectum

Laparotomy is the cornerstone of management and should be recommended even if such evidence as a palpable liver with nodules or shadows in a chest x-ray suggests that secondary spread has already occurred. Excision of the primary is one of the best methods of palliation even if a cure cannot be expected, since it prevents the onset of the distressing symptoms of obstruction or invasion of neighbouring structures such as nerves, ureters, etc.

The subject of large bowel carcinoma causing obstruction is dealt with in Chapter 7. In the absence of obstruction, primary reanastomosis is possible except in very low growths of the rectum where the taking of an adequate margin (about 2 cm) beyond the growth to prevent local recurrence would necessitate sacrificing the anal sphincters. In such circumstances the whole rectum and anal canal is excised, usually by the technique known as *synchronous combined abdominoperineal resection of the rectum* in which two operators work simultaneously, one in the abdomen and one in the perineum with the patient's legs up in the lithotomy position. With sigmoid carcinomas more than 10 cm from the anus it is nearly always possible to take an adequate margin below the growth and preserve the sphincters. Below 10 cm, primary anastomosis becomes increasingly more difficult, especially in the narrow pelvis of the male, but the 'gun', an automatic stapling device, has increased the scope of *restorative* or *anterior resection of the rectum*.

The surgeon removes as much as possible of the lymphatic glandular field which might be expected to drain metastasizing neoplastic cells from the primary. Figure 8.3 shows the areas of peritoneum and length of colon removed for carcinomas at different sites. At present in cases falling into the Dukes' classification as A cases (i.e. the lesion is confined to the mucosa, submucosa and muscle of the colonic wall without having penetrated through to the outer surface of the muscle) the 5-year survival is about 75 per cent, but in B cases (penetrating through the muscle wall) the survival rate falls to about 45 per cent and in C cases (local lymph nodes involved) it is only about 25 per cent. So far no chemotherapeutic or radiotherapeutic regimen has been demonstrated to improve the results. There is, however, some evidence that a combination of radiotherapy and chemotherapy can achieve useful palliation in inoperable cases or in patients in whom metastases occur after operation. An interesting recent advance is the discovery that an antigen called *carcinoembryonic antigen* (CEA) is a good marker for carcinoma of the colon. It is present in the serum of most patients with the disease, disappears after operative resection of the lesion and is reported to reappear in many patients when they develop macroscopic metastases. Some clinics perform a second laparotomy if the CEA becomes positive, in the hope that the recurrences will still be amenable to further surgery.

Diverticular disease

For a discussion of diverticular disease, see p. 113.

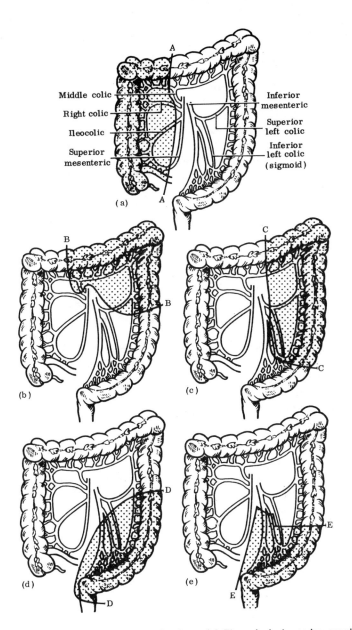

Fig. 8.3 Formal resections of colon. (a) The principal arteries supplying the colon are labelled, although the exact pattern is variable. A—A indicates the limits of excision of a right hemicolectomy. The left branch of the middle colic artery is preserved. If this is not possible, the whole of the transverse colon must be excised, as in (b). (b) B—B represents the limits of excision of a transverse colectomy. The descending branch of the superior left colic artery is preserved. (c) Left hemicolectomy. (d) Anterior resection of the rectum (restorative resection). (e) Radical excision of the rectum (usually a synchronous abdominoperineal approach). Some surgeons advocate that in (c), (d) and (e) the inferior mesenteric artery be tied and divided at its origin from the aorta. (From Hobsley, M. (1979) *Pathways in Surgical Manangement*, Edward Arnold, London)

Ulcerative colitis and Crohn's disease

These two conditions are both of unknown aetiology, and while most of the patients concerned can be assigned without much difficulty to one or the other diagnostic category there are some who seem to lie in a borderland between the two. The importance of this overlap lies in the difficulties of assessing prognosis and selecting the right treatment, and also in the possible aetiological significances—is there a common cause but two characteristic reaction patterns? They are described here as two different conditions, but the overlap should be borne in mind.

Ulcerative colitis
Ulcerative colitis is an inflammatory disease affecting the mucosa of the large bowel—sometimes the whole of it but more often the rectum and the left half only. It is characterized by remissions and exacerbations, by diarrhoea and rectal bleeding, and its onset is mostly in the group aged 15–45 years. It is commoner in Jews than in non-Jews, in white than in black races and in the relatives of sufferers than in the relatives of controls. Psychosomatic factors have received considerable attention but there is little convincing evidence that they are important in causation. Despite the apparently inflammatory nature of the disease, no consistently related micro-organism has been found. It may be an autoimmune disease because there is an association between it and other autoimmune diseases such as systemic lupus erythematosus, uveitis and erythema nodosum and because lymphocytes from sufferers are cytotoxic for cultures of colonic mucosal cells.

Pathology   The condition is confined to the mucosa and submucosa, with infection of the crypts of Lieberkühn progressing to abscess formation being possibly the primary event. The microabscesses may combine to form shallow mucosal ulcers, and the remaining mucosa between ulcers may form pseudopolyps. Attempts at mucosal repair result in vascular granulation tissue, producing both the blood in the faeces and the friable, easily bleeding gut wall that are such characteristic clinical features. Watery diarrhoea is due to mucosal destruction and consequent inability to absorb water and electrolytes. In about 3 per cent of patients the disease is particularly severe and the inflammation extends into the muscle layers and perhaps even to the serosa so that perforation and frank peritonitis may occur ('toxic megacolon').

Diagnosis   The typical sigmoidoscopic features mentioned combined with the barium enema appearances of loss of haustrations with shortening and narrowing of the bowel, are highly suggestive; biopsy via the sigmoidoscope should clinch the diagnosis—but only if other causes of colitis such as amoebiasis and bacillary dysentery can be excluded.

Clinical course   Two-thirds of the patients have a mild form of the disease either intermittent attacks or mild chronic symptoms; their life expectancy is the same as that of the general population. One-quarter have a moderately severe form: individual attacks are severe and require admission to hospital, and there is a definite risk of progression at any moment to the severe category (about 10 per cent) in whom the disease affects the whole wall of the colon. The bowel dilates ('toxic megacolon') and may perforate, but even in the absence of perforation the patient is dangerously ill with fever, severe extracellular depletion from profuse diarrhoea, anaemia, leucocytosis and hypoalbuminaemia. The last-named feature is due to malnutrition in acute-on-chronic cases: acute extracellular depletion itself *increases* plasma protein concentration. The dilated colon is well seen on a plain abdominal x-ray.

Treatment In mild attacks treatment with sulphasalazine 1 g thrice daily is started as a long-term preventive measure of further attacks. Topical steroid treatment as suppositories or retention enemas is the immediate therapy of the present attack. In severe attacks the patient must be admitted to hospital and systemic corticosteroids given in full dosage. When the severe symptoms subside sulphasalazine and retention enemas are added. Should there be a failure to respond and particularly if there is evidence of toxic megacolon or a suspicion of perforation, an emergency operation is necessary. During remission, sulphasalazine should be continued as it seems to be better than steroids at reducing the incidence of relapses. After a patient has had ulcerative colitis for 10 years there is a definite risk of the development of carcinoma of the colon, often multicentric; the risk is particularly marked in the moderate and severe forms and in patients with early onset or with pan-colitis (the whole colon involved). Repeated colonoscopy at frequent intervals with examination of biopsy specimens for dysplastic changes suggesting premalignancy is one form of management. There is also a case for advising prophylactic removal of the colon. The choice lies between total colectomy with a permanent terminal ileostomy on the one hand and subtotal colectomy leaving the rectum *in situ* and performing an ileorectal anastomosis. The rectal stump is still at risk of developing carcinoma but is relatively easy to examine by sigmoidoscopy, and although the faeces are usually watery and defaecation necessarily frequent the patient may prefer this situation to the burden of an ileostomy.

Crohn's disease

This condition can affect any part of the alimentary tract from the mouth to the anus but its most common site is the small bowel, particularly in the distal ileum. In recent years there has been increasing recognition that it also commonly affects the large bowel; such patients have often been misdiagnosed in the past as having ulcerative colitis. Like ulcerative colitis, Crohn's disease is characterized by remissions and relapses and a course that is very variable between one patient and another, it is more common in Jews than in non-Jews and in whites than in blacks, and in relatives of patients than in relatives of controls. Indeed, the coexistence of patients with Crohn's disease and ulcerative colitis in the same family occurs much more often than would be expected by chance. There is an apparently greater incidence in Western than in third-world countries and an increasing incidence with time in Western countries.

An infective aetiology is suggested by the inflammatory nature of the pathology but so far there has been no confirmation of the various candidates mooted such as *Mycobacterium pseudotuberculosis* or various viruses. Psychosomatic factors appear to be even less important in this disease than in ulcerative colitis. Evidence in favour of autoimmunity includes the relationship with systemic manifestations such as polyarthritis, ankylosing spondylitis, eczema and hay fever, the histological similarity of the lesions with those of sarcoidosis and the fact that lymphocytes from some patients have cytotoxic effects on colonic cells growing in tissue culture.

Pathology The naked eye appearances are initially of acute inflammation affecting segments of the bowel of variable length, the red oedematous areas being sharply demarcated at each end from apparently normal bowel and the adjacent mesentery being thickened and containing enlarged fleshy lymph nodes. All layers of the bowel are thickened the mucous membrane may show multiple ulcers and fistula formation is common. The involvement of the serous as well as the other coats of the bowel in the inflammatory process results in adhesions between the affected loop and neighbouring loops of bowel and other viscera; in consequence, fistulae connect with these structures although they often end blindly in intra- or retroperitoneal abscess cavities. The histological features are those of non-specific acute and chronic inflammation but the presence of granulomas, while not essential to the diagnosis is particularly helpful in diagnosing Crohn's disease.

Diagnosis Crohn's disease, like ulcerative colitis, is a non-specific inflammatory disorder of the bowel: there are no diagnostic tests specific for the condition, and specific causes such as bacterial or amoebic dysentery must be excluded by the appropriate investigations—stool culture, sigmoidoscopic biopsy, etc. In half the patients with Crohn's disease affecting the large bowel, the sigmoid colon and rectum are spared; this contrasts with the predilection of ulcerative colitis for the left side of the colon and the rectum. In those patients with sigmoidoscopic evidence of inflammatory disease, biopsy may reveal the typical granulomas without caseation. Radiological appearances are crucial to the clinical diagnosis: opaque enema and then meal examinations may demonstrate cobblestone appearances of the mucosa (due to transverse and longitudinal fissuring of the mucosa with intervening oedematous areas, Fig. 8.4), stricture formation (fibrosis and contracture), spicules of contrast material projecting at right angles from the lumen (the commencement of fistulae) and evidence of bowel obstruction or intraperitoneal masses. Histological material suggesting the diagnosis may be obtained from perianal lesions such as abscesses and fistulae which are commonly encountered in these patients even when the rectum does not appear to be involved, or at laparotomy if one becomes necessary.

Clinical course The predominant symptoms are diarrhoea, usually not bloody, aching central and right lower quadrant abdominal pain with colicky exacerbations, abdominal distension, anorexia, weight loss and lassitude, and nutritional deficiencies (see 'Malabsorption', p. 148). Sometimes the initial onset is acute, with right iliac fossa pain and tenderness and not much diarrhoea; a diagnosis of acute appendicitis is usually made, and on opening the abdomen the appendix and caecum are found to be normal but a variable length of the terminal ileum is bright red and oedematous. The appendix should be removed, since, if the caecum is normal, this procedure does not predispose to fistula formation and the presence of an operative scar in the right iliac fossa would in the future tend to mislead if the appendix had been left in place. Otherwise no active measures are undertaken; this seems a

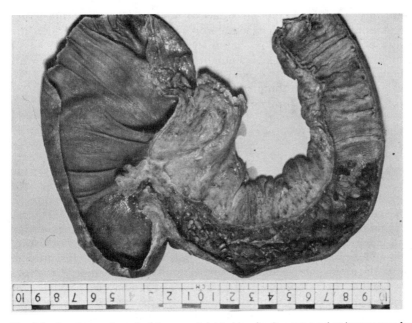

Fig. 8.4 Specimen of terminal ileum and right side of colon removed at laparotomy from a patient with Crohn's disease. The terminal ileum (the most characteristic site) is thickened and the mucosa has the cobblestone appearance typical of Crohn's disease. These features explain why a typical radiological sign in this disease is the 'string sign' in a small bowel opaque meal examination, the ileum narrowing to a long thread-like stricture at its termination and junction with the large bowel. (Specimen by courtesy of the Bland-Sutton Institute of Pathology)

benign form of the disease in that only 1 in 10 of such patients develops further trouble. In most patients, the diagnosis is made radiologically without resort to laparotomy. The prognosis is very uncertain. Some patients get no further trouble after one or two acute episodes, while the general picture is one of gradual deterioration in a number of episodes but on an extremely variable time-scale. Complications include intestinal obstruction, fistula formation (fistulae communicating with the urinary tract are particularly dangerous because of the risk of renal infection), occasionally free perforation into the peritoneal cavity, occasionally rectal blood loss, and rarely carcinoma. There is also a relationship with hepatic disease (usually a mild pericholangitis) and with gallstones (perhaps because the usual disturbance of function of the terminal ileum may produce a deficiency in bile salts by preventing their reabsorption). Related systemic diseases and perineal conditions have been mentioned.

Treatment This is basically medical, although operations become necessary for mechanical complications. Medical treatment includes symptomatic remedies such as codeine or diphenoxylate (Lomotil) for diarrhoea and colic, and periods of intravenous nutrition and nasogastric aspiration for subacute intestinal obstruction, of intravenous feeding for malnutrition due to malabsorption, and of corticosteroids to control episodes of acute inflammatory activity. Azathioprine has its advocates for the acute stage. There is some evidence that long-term sulphasalazine can reduce the incidence of further attacks, but this is less convincing than in the case of ulcerative colitis. When an operation becomes necessary, the segment of bowel responsible for the obstruction, fistula, perforation or bleeding must be removed and intestinal continuity is restored. There is no point in removing all bowel with macroscopic changes of Crohn's disease: such a procedure does not improve the prognosis, and in any case biopsy is likely to demonstrate microscopic changes throughout the gastrointestinal tract.

No diagnosis made

If, after the diagnostic procedures of proctoscopy and sigmoidoscopy, opaque enema and meal, and other special tests already mentioned such as stool culture and rectal biopsy, no definite diagnosis has been reached, the possible lines of action are: to reassure the patient that there is no serious disease present and he is suffering from the so-called irritable bowel syndrome (p. 160); or to ask the patient to return for reassessment and possibly reinvestigation after an interval of time; or to consider the possibility of malabsorption. A decision to reinvestigate means that the clinician thinks it likely that serious disease is present despite the negative results, while a decision to consider malabsorption will depend on specific clinical features of malabsorption or related diseases. In particular, many clinicians feel it is worth while at this stage to ask the patient to avoid milk and milk products for a month in case lactose intolerance—a common specific defect of absorption—is the cause of diarrhoea and abdominal pain.

Malabsorption

Clinical picture

Early symptoms are difficult to assess; they include tiredness and apathy and minor disturbances of bowel habit. A smooth tongue, especially at its lateral borders, may be the only abnormal physical sign at this early stage. In the late stages there is gross loss in weight and the stools are bulky, look pale and greasy, and float on water due to their high content of fat (steatorrhoea). Muscle wasting resulting from protein deficiency and catabolism is associated with the pot-belly of hypoalbuminaemic ascites, the hypoalbuminaemia being due not only to lack of protein but also to loss of albumin from the damaged mucosa of the bowel. Specific vitamin deficiencies include hyperkeratosis of skin (vitamin A), a bleeding diathesis (K), macrocytic anaemia (B_{12} and folic acid), paraesthesiae, skeletal pain and tetany (D—and also calcium lack), and the smooth red tongue, cracked lips, dermatitis and peripheral neuropathy of the rest of the vitamin B complex. Iron deficiency also produces anaemia, of the hypochromic microcytic variety. Physical signs include those of the above conditions plus clubbing of the nail-beds and hyperactive bowel sounds.

Is malabsorption present?

The most commonly used test is the quantitative measurement of fat in the faeces on a standard diet (p. 46).

Does the radiological evidence help?

Opaque meal and enema examinations may have demonstrated anatomical abnormalities that can produce malabsorption (e.g. operations such as partial gastrectomy and gastrojejunostomy; congenital lesions such as reduplications; or acquired lesions such as a gastrocolic fistula).

These conditions produce malabsorption by reducing the time for which the food is in contact with the small bowel absorptive mucosa—either by anatomical diversion or by an increased rate of transit—or by encouraging the growth in the small bowel of large bowel organisms which split the conjugated bile salts and thereby prevent their reabsorption in the terminal ileum so that they are lost in the faeces.

Rapid transit

The anatomical abnormality may be so obviously the cause of malabsorption that its surgical correction is indicated without further ado. This is the situation with a gastrocolic fistula, which usually arises either from a carcinoma of the transverse colon spreading into the stomach or from a recurrent ulcer of the jejunal loop, after an inadequate operation for peptic ulcer, penetrating both into stomach and into colon. The obvious explanation for malabsorption, complete bypass of the small intestine, is probably too simple; an opaque meal usually fails to demonstrate the fistula but an opaque enema does, so the flow of material is probably from the colon into the stomach, presumably because the pressure in the colon is higher. The probable mechanism is thus colonization of the stomach and small intestine with large bowel fauna.

Should the abnormality shown be less obviously responsible for the malabsorption, it might be thought advisable to demonstrate rapid intestinal transit. After vagotomy or partial gastrectomy, rapid gastric emptying is associated with rapid transit of the meal through the small intestine, a hypertonic glucose meal reaching the terminal ileum within 5 minutes of ingestion; thus objective evidence of rapid emptying and associated symptoms of the dumping syndrome (Chapter 5) constitute sufficient evidence of intestinal hurry. Techniques to quantify intestinal hurry are available: non-absorbable radio-opaque markers given by mouth can be collected in the faeces to give a measure of overall transit time, while a more elegant system uses radiotelemetering pressure-sensitive capsules as markers. The position of these capsules, which contain chromium-51, can be determined with the aid of an external scintillation counter; because their localization in the stomach, jejunum or ileum can be deduced from the nature of the pressure record they broadcast, the rate of transit can be determined separately in different portions of the alimentary tract.

Bacterial colonization of small intestine

Bacteria growing in the small intestine interfere with the normal mechanisms of absorption by competition and doubtless by altering various characteristics of the medium such as pH. A good test of such colonization is the bile acid breath test. Bile acids conjugated with glycine or taurine are excreted in the bile and normally are almost completely absorbed in the terminal ileum (Sanford: *Digestive System Physiology*, Chapter 4)—the enterohepatic circulation. However, if exposed to large bowel bacteria, deconjugation occurs and the glycine or taurine is metabolized, with the formation of CO_2. If the patient ingests bile acid conjugated with ^{14}C-labelled glycine, the appearance of ^{14}C-labelled CO_2 in the breath signifies abnormal exposure of the intestinal bile acid to micro-organisms, either because of their overgrowth in the small intestine or because of failure of reabsorption normally in the terminal ileum—for example, because of surgical excision of that part of the bowel, or because its functions have been impaired by local pathology such as Crohn's disease.

Is the fault in the intestinal wall?

If the luminal factors of hurry, diversion or bacterial colonization are not suggested by the radiological evidence, then the two important remaining groups are the other luminal factor of pancreatic exocrine insufficiency or defects in the absorptive processes within the wall of the intestinal mucosa. The latter are easier to test than the former, using, for example, the xylose absorption/excretion test. Xylose, a five-carbon sugar, is relatively poorly absorbed, but its absorption is not at all dependent on pancreatic enzymes. If intestinal absorption is normal, at least 4 g should be recoverable from the urine during the 5 hours after the ingestion of 25 g, and blood levels should reach 20 mg/dl during the second hour after ingestion.

Tests for pancreatic function are described in Chapter 3. If the xylose test suggests, however, that intestinal function is at fault, other tests can be undertaken to try further to categorize the defect.

Vitamin B_{12} absorption test

This test depends upon the fact that the vitamin B_{12}–intrinsic factor complex can be absorbed only in the terminal ileum. The body stores of the vitamin are first saturated with an intramuscular injection of 1 mg, and a dose labelled with a radioactive marker is then ingested. Urine is collected for the next 24 hours, and should contain at least 7 per cent of the radioactivity if absorption is normal. If absorption is abnormally low, the function of the terminal ileum is abnormal, or the patient lacks intrinsic factor or there is an interference with absorption due to bacterial overgrowth. The latter two possibilities can be examined by repeating the test either with the addition of exogenous intrinsic factor or after a course of appropriate antibiotics.

Peroral intestinal mucosal biopsy

Specimens of the mucosa of the duodenum or upper jejunum can be obtained either with biopsy forceps via an endoscope or with the Crosby–Kugler capsule. The capsule is passed on the end of a long tube and, after it has negotiated the pylorus, its passage is followed radiologically. When it reaches the biopsy site, a piece of jejunal mucosa is sucked into the capsule by negative pressure applied via the tube and cut off to lie within the capsule by a guillotine that is also activated by the observer. The capsule is then withdrawn, and the specimen examined histologically and also, where appropriate, by biochemical techniques.

The important biochemical deficiency is that of disaccharidases, since these enzymes are confined to the brush border of the epithelial cells. Absence of an enzyme can be confirmed by a breath test. Since no mammalian cell can produce hydrogen but large gut micro-organisms can do so by the fermentation of carbohydrate, giving lactose to a patient with the commonest disaccharidase deficiency, alactasia, results in the appearance of hydrogen in the breath when the unabsorbed lactose reaches the intestine.

Most of the other conditions producing malabsorption by interfering with intestinal mucosal function can be diagnosed from the histological appearances. These include the sprue complex of diseases, lymphoma, lymphangiectasia, hypogammaglobulinaemia, dermatitis herpetiformis, non-granulomatous jejunitis, Whipple's disease and parasitic infestations. The less uncommon of these conditions are described below, but it is interesting that iatrogenic causes such as post-x-irradiation changes, and massive bowel resections are now among the more common causes. (For details of disturbances of transport of non-electrolytes, see Sanford: *Digestive System Physiology*, Chapter 4.)

Coeliac disease (sprue)
This disease has a large number of synonyms, including 'non-tropical sprue' and 'idiopathic steatorrhoea'. It is best defined as a tendency towards, or actual presence of, malabsorption for all food components associated with a characteristic change in mucosal histology and a prompt clinical improvement when gluten-containing cereals are withdrawn from the diet. While the symptoms and signs of malabsorption usually occur when the infant is started on cereals, many patients only present for the first time in adulthood and it is certain that the condition may exist in subclinical form for many years.

How gluten, the water-insoluble protein of certain cereal grains, damages the intestine is unknown. Flour made from wheat, barley or rye is toxic to all susceptible individuals, from oats to some of them. Typical symptoms of distension, colicky pain, diarrhoea and malaise are produced within a few hours of exposure in a sufferer who has hitherto been on a gluten-free diet. The characteristic histological appearances are a loss of the normal villi, leaving a flat mucosa, a reduction in the number and gross morphological changes in the absorptive cells, and an infiltration of the lamina propria with plasma cells and lymphocytes. Studies of the enzymes of the absorptive cells show deficiencies of many kinds. Withdrawal of gluten from the diet leads, within a few weeks, to a restitution of normal appearances and biochemical properties and the relief of symptoms.

Treatment consists of maintenance on a gluten-free diet, and the prognosis is generally excellent. There is an increased risk of malignancy, particularly of lymphomas, in these patients. There is also an interesting relationship between coeliac disease and a skin disease, dermatitis herpetiformis. All patients with the latter probably have at least a mild form of coeliac disease but only a few patients with clinical coeliac disease have dermatitis herpetiformis.

Tropical sprue

Unlike coeliac disease, tropical sprue is not a clear-cut entity but probably a group of conditions producing malabsorption in association with histological changes in the intestinal mucosa. There is some flattening of the villi, but not as completely as in coeliac disease. While it is endemic in many parts of the tropics, it can also occur in epidemic form. It was originally thought that tropical sprue only affected foreigners from temperate climes who were living in the tropics, but it is now known to affect the indigenous as well. The fiction that coeliac disease did not occur in the tropics has also been disproved. Moreover, many conditions rife in hot countries, including bacillary dysentery and parasitic diseases such as amoebiasis, giardiasis and strongyloidiasis, not to mention tuberculous enteritis, can also cause chronic diarrhoea and malabsorption. Thus the diagnosis at present is really a matter of excluding these other conditions and finding stunted villi.

Treatment is empirical: diarrhoea is controlled with opiates or diphenoxylate (Lomotil), deficiencies produced by malabsorption are corrected and courses of antibiotics have been tried with variable results. Deficiency of folate is a marked feature, and treatment with folate rapidly makes the patient feel better.

Whipple's disease

This interesting uncommon disease of males always involves the duodenojejunal junction, can also involve practically any other tissue or organ including joints, pleurae, lung, heart and central nervous system, and is always associated with a high erythrocyte sedimentation rate. Common presentations include pyrexia, arthralgia, enlarged lymph nodes, endocarditis, muscle wasting and skin pigmentation, with or without the features of malabsorption.

The histological appearances of the affected tissues are specific for the disease: there is infiltration with large foamy macrophages containing numerous granules of glycoprotein that stain with the periodic acid–Schiff (PAS) stain, together with an abundance of many small bacilli (only 1–2.5 μm in length, but easily visible with electron microscopy). Thus, in patients presenting with malabsorption the diagnosis is usually made by intestinal biopsy.

This condition used to be uniformly fatal, but relatively recently it has been shown that treatment with antibiotics—not necessarily broad-spectrum (even penicillin alone has had its reported successes)—cures the clinical manifestations with disappearance of the organisms from the tissues.

Parasitic diseases

Parasitic infestation of the intestine with consequent symptoms must be one of the commonest causes of gastroenterological disease. Poor sanitation, crowded

Table 8.1 Intestinal parasites

	Protozoa		Roundworms (helminths)		
Disease and/or organism	Giardia lamblia	Coccidiosis Isospora belli, I. hominis, I. natalensis	Ascariasis Ascaris lumbricoides	Strongyloidiasis Strongyloides stercoralis	Ancylostomiasis (hookworm) Ancylostoma duodenale, Necator americanus
Distribution	World-wide	World-wide	World-wide	Warm, moist areas; faecal contamination of soil	Warm, moist areas; faecal contamination of soil
Incidence of disease	2–30%	Very variable; common in Africa, Middle East and South America	Common in tropics	Common in tropics	Common in tropics
Intermediate host	None required	None required	None required	None required	None required
Morphological forms	Cyst Trophozoite	Sporulated oöcyst, sporozoites, trophozoites, etc.	Ova, larvae, adult worms 20 cm long	Rhabditoid larvae (free living); filariform larvae (infective, can penetrate skin and buccal mucosa)	Ova in faeces develop in soil into rhabditoid larvae → filariform larvae (infective, can penetrate skin and buccal mucosa)
Infection route	Ingestion of cysts	Ingestion of oöcysts	Ingestion of eggs	See above	See above
Location	Duodenum and proximal small bowel	Duodenum and small bowel	Ova → larvae in duodenum → portal veins → lungs (pneumonitis) → bronchi → pharynx → swallowed → adult small intestinal worms	→ circulation to lungs → alveoli → trachea and pharynx → swallowed → infection of whole gastrointestinal tract → eggs → rhabditoid larvae → faeces	→ circulation to lungs → alveoli → trachea and pharynx → swallowed → become attached to duodenal mucosa

Table 8.1 cont.

	Protozoa		Roundworms (helminths)		
Clinical	Asymptomatic Malabsorption as in coeliac sprue Epidemic diarrhoea Travellers' diarrhoea	Acute fever, headache Diarrhoea, weight loss, colic Steatorrhoea. Self-limiting (less than 6 months)	Hypersensitivity reactions Obstruction: intestinal obstruction, acute appendicitis, obstructive jaundice Malabsorption by competition	Petechiae, rashes, oedema and urticaria Pneumonitis, asthma, fever, dyspnoea, haemoptysis. Weight loss, anorexia, colic, vomiting, diarrhoea, steatorrhoea, jaundice, intestinal obstruction Death	Iron-deficiency anaemia (mechanical loss plus ingestion by worms). Hypoproteinaemia, ?malabsorption (by competition) – but probably not. Anorexia or increased appetite Rarely, pneumonitis, pruritis
Diagnosis	Duodenal mucosal biopsy (Masson's stain). (Examination of faeces often negative)	Duodenal, mucosal biopsy (Examination of faeces often negative)	Eosinophilia Examination of faeces for worms, sputum for larvae. Opaque meal x-ray studies	Eosinophilia Larvae in stools Examination of duodenal secretions	Iron-deficiency anaemia Folic acid deficiency Eosinophilia. Eggs in faeces. Mucosal biopsy and duodenal secretions
Treatment	Metronidazole (Flagyl)	No specific available	Piperazine citrate	Thiabendazole	Bephenium

Table 8.1 cont.

| | Flatworms | | | | |
| | Tapeworms (cestodes) | | | Flukes (trematodes) | |
Disease and/or organism	*Diphyllobothrium latum*	*Taenia solium*	*Taenia saginata*	Giant intestinal fluke (*Fasciolopsis buski*)	*Clonorchis sinensis*
Distribution	World-wide	World-wide	World-wide	Far East	Far East
Incidence of disease	Common where raw fish is eaten (e.g. Japan, the Arctic)	Common	Common	—	—
Intermediate host	Fish	Pig	Cattle	Snails	Fish
Morphological forms	Adult 3–10 m long, hermaphrodite; scolex (head) anchors worm to intestinal mucosa of host; ova	Larvae (cysticerci); oncospheres; adult worm 1–3 m, hermaphrodite	Adult 4–25 m, hermaphrodite; ova in faeces; larvae (cysticerci)	Adult ovoid worms (20–75 mm long); ova in human and swine faeces; larvae, (cercariae) in snails, become cysts on plants	Adult worms; ova; cysts in fish
Infection route	Ingestion of infected raw fish	Ingestion of infected raw or undercooked pork	Ingestion of infected or uncooked beef	Ingestion of raw water plants	Ingestion of raw fish

Table 8.1 cont

| | Flatworms | | | | |
	Tapeworms (cestodes)			Flukes (trematodes)	
Location	Ileum; less often jejunum, colon	Cysticercosis can affect every tissue and organ: this can occur if ova are ingested whereupon oncospheres can penetrate intestinal wall and spread by blood vessels	Small intestine: the scolex evaginates from the cysticercus in the duodenum and attaches to intestinal wall. Eggs are eaten by cattle, larvae hatch in duodenum, penetrate wall of intestine and spread by blood vessels (cysticercosis)	Larvae emerge from cysts in duodenum, become fixed to small intestinal mucosa. Mechanical intestinal obstruction, haemorrhages, and abscesses may result	Larvae develop from ingested cysts in duodenum. By unknown route they reach the biliary passages where they stay
Clinical	Vitamin B_{12} deficiency by competition. Occasionally, mechanical bowel obstruction	Adult worm usually symptomless. Cysticercosis symptoms depend on site; greatly exacerbated when the larvae die	Malnutrition (by competition), diarrhoea, loss in weight, abdominal colic. Intestinal obstruction. Acute appendicitis. Human cysticercosis is rare	Diarrhoea and hunger pains. Oedema and ascites. Prostration and death	Adenomatous change and fibrosis in bile ducts, proceeding sometimes to cholangio-carcinoma. Obstructive jaundice and ascending cholangitis
Diagnosis	Eosinophilia. If B_{12} deficiency, macrocytic anaemia and megaloblastic bone marrow. Ova or segments in faeces	Eosinophilia. Ova (identical with *Taenia saginata*) and typical gravid proglottides (segments) in stools Excision-biopsy of cysticerci	Eosinophilia. Ova in faeces (identical with *Taenia solium*) Typical gravid proglottides	Leucocytosis and eosinophilia. Ova in faeces	Eosinophilia. Ova in faeces
Treatment	Niclosamide	Mepacrine hydrochloride	Niclosamide	Hexyl resorcinol	Emetine, then chloro-quine

For schistosomiasis (*Schistosoma japonicum*, *S. mansoni* and *S. haematobium*, see Chapter 6.

living conditions and close associations with any animal host involved are all predisposing factors, the most important being poor health-education. A table of the important features of the commoner parasites, their life cycle and the diseases they produce is given (Table 8.1). The organisms known to be associated with the picture of intestinal malabsorption are *Giardia lamblia*, coccidiosis, *Strongyloides stercoralis* and *Ancylostoma duodenale*. All these can be diagnosed by examination of aspirate or mucosal biopsy from the intestine.

Intestinal bypass operations for morbid obesity

Morbid obesity can be defined as an increase in weight to at least twice the ideal for the patient. This is becoming an increasing problem in North America and, to a lesser extent, in Europe.

The serious consequences of gross obesity in terms of medical disease—death rates in people under the age of 40 years are at least doubled—and of physical, social and psychological handicaps are so great that, when conservative measures of dieting or controlled starvation fail, a surgical operation may be advised.

The most commonly used procedure in the past has been some form of jejunoileal bypass, preserving the bypassed loop of bowel so that it can be used to restore the normal anatomy and physiology if the sequelae are too severe for the patient to tolerate. About the first 35 cm of proximal jejunum is anastomosed end-to-end to the terminal 10 cm of the ileum, while the intervening long loop of jejunoileum is closed at its proximal end and anastomosed at its distal end to the transverse colon. Note that this procedure preserves not only the terminal ileum but also that important structure, the ileocaecal valve (Sanford: *Digestive System Physiology*, Chapter 6). Operations reducing gastric capacity are becoming more popular.

The effects of all these operations are similar. Weight loss is rapid at first (about 5 kg per month) but after 6 months more gradual until a plateau is reached—usually rather above and never below the patient's ideal weight. Abdominal distension and colicky pain, diarrhoea and steatorrhoea are the usual symptoms, and malabsorption of most dietary components can be demonstrated although the retention of the terminal ileum tends to keep vitamin B_{12} absorption normal. The most serious of the possible long-term complications is cirrhosis, the mechanism of its production probably being protein malnutrition. A worsening of the picture of malabsorption can be due to bacterial overgrowth in the bypassed loop, and this responds to antibiotics.

Short bowel syndrome

Massive resection of the small bowel results in malabsorption through the loss of mucosal absorptive surface. Causes for such resection include gangrene induced by involvement of the bowel in a volvulus or hernia with consequent strangulation, or widespread disease such as Crohn's regional enteritis. The severity of the malabsorption and details of the dietary constituents most affected depend on the length of small bowel remaining and also on its anatomical site, i.e. whether proximal or distal. Patients rarely survive if they are left with less than 60 cm of small bowel (as well as the duodenum), and the effects of any loss including the terminal ileum are greater than those of the loss of the same length but not including the terminal ileum because of the localization of the absorption of bile salts and of vitamin B_{12} to that region.

Two other effects of massive intestinal resection are the formation of oxalate stones in the renal tract and an increase in the maximal capacity of the stomach to secrete acid. The mechanism of the stone formation is that unabsorbed fatty acids in the intestinal lumen combine with dietary calcium, thereby reducing the amount of calcium available to bind oxalate ions as insoluble oxalate: the oxalate is absorbed instead, producing oxaluria and hence the calculi. The mechanism of the hypersecretion is unknown, but it seems possible that it involves an interference with the metabolism of gastrin; one of the normal sites for the breakdown of gastrin is the intestinal mucosa.

Operations to delay the transit of food along the short intestine have been described (e.g. reversed loops or recycling circuits) but have largely proved ineffectual. Management is therefore via dietary control. At first the patient is given nothing by mouth and nutrition is maintained by the intravenous route—intravenous feeding or alimentation. When diarrhoea subsides to manageable proportions (less than 2 litres per 24 hours) after a few months, intravenous feeding is continued but oral feeding cautiously introduced. After 6–12 months, absorption gradually improves by poorly understood mucosal adaptations so that ultimately most patients with 20 per cent of small bowel remaining can manage on an entirely oral intake of food (apart, of course, from vitamin B_{12}).

Intravenous feeding

The maintenance of a patient in normal nutritional balance entirely by the intravenous route requires a sound knowledge of the basic physiological principles. The total number of non-protein calories must be sufficient to meet the energy requirements of a patient in whom recent trauma or surgery or such factors as sepsis and pyrexia increase the demands above the baseline of about 8400 MJ (2000 kcal) per 24 hours. This energy can be provided as carbohydrate or as fat, but if fat is used it should not contribute more than two-thirds of the non-protein energy, the rest being carbohydrate; otherwise, ketosis will occur.

Carbohydrate is usually given as hypertonic solutions of glucose, say 2.78 mol/l (50 g/dl), or ten times the tonicity of plasma, otherwise the necessary calorie intake would only be achieved with the disadvantage of giving an excessive intake of water; by introducing them into large volumes of blood circulating in such vessels as the superior vena cava, the hypertonic solutions can be rapidly diluted as soon as they enter the circulation so that they do not cause haemolysis. Fat is available as emulsions (e.g. of soyabean oil) which are isotonic and can be infused into peripheral veins. Although energy can be satisfactorily provided by carbohydrate alone, lack of the essential fatty acids on such a regimen leads to a scaly dermatitis after some days. Protein is given either as hydrolysates of casein or fibrin, or as solutions

Table 8.2 A regimen of intravenous feeding

Time	Line A	Line B
08.00–16.00	Synthamin 9* (synthetic amino acids) 500 ml	50% dextrose 1 litre‡
		+ Multibionta (vitamins of B group)
16.00–00.00	20% Intralipid+ (fat emulsion) 500 ml	at 40 ml per hour via Burette
00.00–08.00	Synthamin 9 500 ml	

Notes

General Write times on prescription as above.
Lines A and B run simultaneously, using a Y-type giving-set designed for the purpose.
Line B requires a set with a burette chamber, e.g. a Soluset.
It should be noted that routine blood samples will not be taken within 8 hours of infusing Intralipid. Urine must be tested for glucose 4-hourly; added insulin may be needed and glycosuria rapidly results in fluid depletion.

Specific *Higher, or lower, strength Synthamin (Travenol) solutions may be used. Other preparations using crystalline L-form amino acids are also suitable. Electrolyte-free solutions are available and may be required in special circumstances; e.g. renal or hepatic failure.

+Use 10% Intralipid initially and change after 4–5 days to 20%. Check plasma daily for turbidity. Patients with hepatic impairment: give only 500 ml 10% Intralipid alternate days. Fat-soluble vitamin preparations are available which may be added to Intralipid.

‡Trace elements (commercially available; e.g. Addamel (KabiVitrum) containing Ca 5 mmol, Mg 1.5 mmol, Fe^{3+} 50 μmol, Zn 20 μmol, Mn 40 μmol, Cu^{2+} 5 μmol, fluoride 50 μmol, iodide 1 μmol and Cl 13.3 mmol, in 10 ml) should be added to the 50% dextrose. Some patients will also require extra KCl in this line, especially if insulin is added. These additions are ideally done in pharmacy. Insulin is best given via constant infusion pump.

Fat-soluble vitamins (e.g. Vitlipid (KabiVitrum), a preparation of vitamins A, D_2 and K_1) are given mixed with the fat emulsion in a dose of 1 vial daily.

Vitamins Folic acid should be given intramuscularly once a week (folate stores are large, but not readily utilized in severely ill patients). B_{12} should be given monthly (it is safe, and protects against unmasking B_{12} deficiency by giving folate).

Calories The regimen shown gives approximately 12.6 MJ (3000 kcal) per day in 2.5 litres. Once parenteral nutrition is well established and obligatory water retention passed, the 50% dextrose can be increased to 60 ml per hour, giving 16.8 MJ (4000 kcal) in 3 litres; at the same time a more concentrated amino acid solution can be introduced.

of synthetic L-amino acids. About 120–150 g per day of amino acids should be an adequate quantity, even in patients with a catabolic state. Water and electrolyte requirements are discussed on p. 000, but phosphate is required to the extent of about 50 mmol per day, and calcium, magnesium, the trace elements (zinc, copper, manganese, cobalt) and the vitamins also require consideration. For obvious reasons of the differences between patients and clinical situations it is impossible to generalize, but Table 8.2 sets out detailed instructions for one possible regimen and gives some idea of the complexities involved in trying to replace the lost function of absorption by the gastrointestinal tract.

Irritable bowel

In many patients the diagnostic endeavour, no matter how enthusiastically pursued, draws blank and no organic disease can be demonstrated. It is at this stage that the label 'irritable bowel' or one of its many synonyms (such as 'irritable colon', 'spastic colitis', 'mucous colitis' and many others) is applied to the patient.

This label is in no sense diagnostic, but it is most useful with regard to management since it implies that unless the clinical situation changes no further effort is to be made by the clinician to unearth an organic cause for the complaints and that treatment should be symptomatic.

The ease and certainty with which this diagnosis is reached depend on how clearly the clinician elicits a link between periods of marked symptoms and emotional stress. In all of us bowel function is to some extent affected by worry fear and tension: students who have had an attack of diarrhoea on the morning of an important academic examination have experienced this phenomenon. The more clear-cut such a relationship, the earlier can the diagnostic procedures be abandoned, but if serious mistakes are not to occur then the clinician must be experienced.

Patients with the irritable bowel syndrome tend to fall into three groups: those with lower abdominal pain, usually with constipation; those with diarrhoea, usually painless; and those with alternating constipation and diarrhoea (and particularly in these a colonic neoplasm must be excluded). Bloating with gaseous distension is common in all three types. Special measurements of colonic intraluminal pressure and of motility have demonstrated abnormalities of pattern compared with control subjects, and even relationships between the severity of these abnormalities and emotional stress. However, the methods of investigation are not readily available, or readily applicable, in clinical circumstances. Treatment thus resolves itself into an explanation that nothing organic is amiss, a sympathetic discussion of the link between the patient's symptoms and his psyche, and dietary and pharmacological remedies for the symptoms.

For patients with pain and constipation, increasing the bulk and water content of the stools with a high residue diet including particularly plenty of bran (Sanford: *Digestive System Physiology*, Chapter 6) is the most generally successful advice. For diarrhoea, opiates should be avoided because they increase bowel spasm and tend to be addictive; the most useful preparations are diphenoxylate (Lomotil) and loperamide (Imodium).

Despite all the recent advances in gastroenterology referred to in previous pages, it is a sad truth that the largest single category of patients consulting a gastroenterologist in the Western world today consists of people in this group of the irritable bowel syndrome, of unknown aetiology and empirical (and uncertain) treatment.

Further reading

Alexander-Williams, J. (1976). Crohn's disease and the surgeon. In *Current Surgical Practice,* vol. 1, pp. 192–201. Ed. by G. J. Hadfield and M. Hobsley. Edward Arnold, London.

Arseculeratne, S. N., Panabokke, R. G. and Navaratnam, C. (1980). Pathogenesis of necrotising enteritis with special reference to intestinal hypersensitivity reactions. *Gut* **21,** 265–278.

Burkitt, D. P. (1971). Epidemiology of cancer of the colon and rectum. *Cancer* **28,** 3–13.

Cameron, A. (1975). Left colon resection. *British Journal of Hospital Medicine* **17,** 281–289.

Cobden, I., Rothwell, J. and Axon, A. T. R. (1980). Intestinal permeability and screening tests for coeliac disease. *Gut* **21,** 512–518.

Compston, J. E. and Creamer, B. (1977). The consequences of small intestinal resection. *Quarterly Journal of Medicine* **46,** 485–497.

Hawley, P. R. (1978). Common anal conditions. In *Current Surgical Practice,* vol. 2, pp. 87–110. Ed. by G. J. Hadfield and M. Hobsley. Edward Arnold, London.

Higgins, G. A. Jr (1978). The pros and cons of irradiation treatment of colorectal cancer. *Surgical Annual* **10,** 175–190.

International Agency for Research on Cancer: Intestinal Microecology Group. (1977). Dietary fibre, transit time, faecal bacteria, steroids and colon cancer in two Scandinavian populations. *Lancet* **ii,** 207–211.

Langman, M. J. S. (1976). *The Epidemiology of Chronic Digestive Disease.* Edward Arnold, London.

Lennard-Jones, J. E. (1976). Ulcerative Colitis. In *Current Surgical Practice,* vol. 1, pp. 185–191. Ed. by G. J. Hadfield and M. Hobsley. Edward Arnold, London.

Marsden, P. D. (Ed.) (1978). *Intestinal Parasites. Clinics in Gastroenterology* **7,** no. 1.

Morson, B. C. and Dawson, I. M. P. (1972). *Gastrointestinal Pathology.* Blackwell Scientific, Oxford.

Phillip, S. F. (1972). Diarrhea: a current view of the pathophysiology. *Gastroenterology* **63,** 495–518.

Russell, R. I. (1980). Intravenous nutrition and elemental diets. In *Scientific Foundations of Gastroenterology,* pp. 130–140. Ed. by W. Sircus and A. N. Smith. Heinemann Medical, London.

Silk, D. B. A. (1980). Small intestine: disordered protein metabolism. In *Scientific Foundations of Gastroenterology,* pp. 408–425. Ed. by W. Sircus and A. N. Smith. Heinemann Medical, London.

Taylor, I., Basu, P., Hammond, P., Darby, C. and Flynn, M. (1980). Effect of bile acid perfusion on colonic motor function in patients with the irritable colon syndrome. *Gut* **21,** 843–847.

Taylor, I., Rowling, J. and West, C. (1979). Adjuvant cytotoxic liver perfusion for colorectal cancer. *British Journal of Surgery* **66,** 833–837.

Thomson, J. P. S. (1978). Anorectal prolapse. In *Current Surgical Practice,* vol. 2, pp. 66–76. Ed. by G. J. Hadfield and M. Hobsley. Edward Arnold, London.

Appendix

Approved drug names and proprietary preparations in the UK and in the USA

United Kingdom		United States of America	
Approved name	Common proprietary preparations	Approved name	Common proprietary preparations
Acetylsalicylic acid	Aspirin	Acetylsalicylic acid	Aspirin
Aluminium hydroxide	Aludrox Gelusil	Aluminium hydroxide	Aludrox Gelusil
Ampicillin	Penbritin Pentrexyl Vidopen	Ampicillin	Alpen Amcill Omnipen Penbritin Polycillin Principen Totacillin
Aprotinin	Trasylol	Aprotinin	Trasylol
Atropine methonitrate	Eumydrin	Atropine methonitrate	Metropine
Azathioprine	Imuran	Azathioprine	Imuran
Bephenium	Alcopar	Bephenium	—
Carbenoxolone	Biogastrone Duogastrone	Carbenoxolone	Biogastrone Duogastrone
Chenodeoxycholic acid	Chendol	Chenodeoxycholic acid	Chenix
Chloramphenicol	Chloromycetin	Chloramphenicol	Chloromycetin Amphicol Mychel

United Kingdom		United States of America	
Approved name	Common proprietary preparations	Approved name	Common proprietary preparations
Chloroquine	Avloclor Nivaquine	Chloroquine	Aralen Roquine
Chlorpromazine	Largactil	Chlorpromazine	Largactil Thorazine
Cholestyramine	Questran	Cholestyramine	Cuemid Questran
Cimetidine	Tagamet	Cimetidine	Tagamet
Clofibrate	Atromid-S	Clofibrate	Atromid-S
Dextropropoxyphene	Distalgesic	Propoxyphene	Darvon
Diphenoxylate	Lomotil	Diphenoxylate	Lomotil
Emetine hydrochloride	—	Emetine hydrochloride	—
5-Fluorouracil	Fluoro-uracil	Fluorouracil	Efudex Fluoroplex
Gentamicin	Cidomycin Genticin	Gentamicin	Garamycin
Halothane	Fluothane	Halothane	Fluothane
Hexylresorcinol	Sucrets	Hexylresorcinol	Crystoids
Indomethacin	Indocin	Indomethacin	Indocin
Iopanoic acid	Telepaque	Iopanoic acid	Telepaque
Isoniazid	Rimifon	Isoniazid	INH Niconyl Nydrazid
Lactulose	Duphalac	Lactulose	Cephulac
Lignocaine	Xylocaine	Lidocaine	Xylocaine
Loperamide	Imodium	Loperamide	Imodium
Mepacrine hydrochloride	Quinacrine	Quinacrine hydrochloride	Atabrine hydrochloride

United Kingdom		United States of America	
Approved name	Common proprietary preparations	Approved name	Common proprietary preparations
Mepyramine maleate	Anthisan	Pyrilamine maleate	Anthisan
Methylcellulose	Cologel	Methylcellulose	Methocel
Metronidazole	Flagyl	Metronidazole	Flagyl
Mitomycin	Mitomycin C	Mitomycin	Mutamycin
Neomycin	Mycifradin Nivemycin	Neomycin	Mycifradin Neobiotic
Niclosamide	Yomesan	Niclosamide	—
Niridazole	Ambilhar	Niridazole	Ambilhar
Paracetamol	Calpol Panadol Panasorb	Acetaminophen	Apamide Nebs Tempra Tylenol
Pentagastrin	Peptavol	Pentagastrin	Peptavol
Phenobarbitone	Gardenal Luminal	Phenobarbital	Luminal
Phenylbutazone	Butazolidin	Phenylbutazone	Butazolidin
Pilocarpine nitrate	—	Pilocarpine nitrate	—
Piperazine citrate	Antepar	Piperazine citrate	Antepar Multifuge Vermizine
Sodium antimonylgluconate	—	Sodium antimonylgluconate	—
Sulphasalazine	Salazopyrine	Sulfasalazine, Salazosulfapyridine	Azulfidine Rorasul
Testosterone	Sustanon	Testosterone	Androlin Andronaq Malestrone Neo-Hombreol Oreton
Thiabendazole	Mintezol	Thiabendazole	Mintezol

United Kingdom		United States of America	
Approved name	Common proprietary preparations	Approved name	Common proprietary preparations
Ursodeoxycholic acid	Urso	—	—
Vancomycin	Vancocin	Vancomycin	Vancocin
Vasopressin	Pitressin	Vasopressin	Pitressin
Vitamin K:		Vitamin K:	
K_1	Synkavit	K_1	Mephyton
(Phytomenadione)	Konakion	Phytonadione	
		Phylloquinone	
		Phytomenadione	
K_3	Menadione	K_3 Menadione	
	Menaphthone	Menaphthone	
		Menadiol sodium	Synkavite
		diphosphate	Kappadione

Index

Index